CORONARY ANGIOGRAPHY

An Introduction
to Interpretation and Technique

CORONARY ANGIOGRAPHY

An Introduction
to Interpretation and Technique

James F. Silverman, M.D.

Associate Dean for Clinical Affairs
Professor of Diagnostic Radiology
Stanford University School of Medicine

Chief of Staff
Stanford University Hospital
Stanford, California

To my wife Barbara and my children, Andrew, Ben, and Susan (who inspired the heart model) and to Drs. Walter Rohlfing, Charles Kilhenny, and Jack Lawson, for their encouragement along the way.

Sponsoring Editor: Katharine Pitcoff
Developmental Editor and
 Production Coordinator: Susan Harrington
Book Designer: Lisa Mirski
Cover Designer: Leigh McLellan
Cover Photographer: William Thompson

Library of Congress Cataloging in Publication Data

Silverman, James F.
 Coronary angiography.

 Includes bibliographies and index.
 1. Angiography. 2. Coronary arteries—Radiography.
I. Title. [DNLM: 1. Coronary Vessels—radiography.
WG 300 S587c]
RC683.5.A5S56 1984   616.1′2306572   84-11036
ISBN 0-201-07148-7
 DEFGHIJ-MA-898

We are indebted to the following authors and publications for permission to reprint photographs and line art from previously published articles.

Figure 1-2: Adapted from an original painting by Frank H. Netter, M.D., from THE CIBA COLLECTION OF MEDICAL ILLUSTRATIONS, copyright © by CIBA Pharmaceutical Company, Division of CIBA-GEIGY Corporation.

Figures 1-5 and 1-8: Courtesy of Donald Baim, M.D.

Figures 1-9, 1-10, 1-11, and 1-12: Abrams, H. L. and D. F. Adams. 1969. The coronary arteriogram: Structural and functional aspects. *NEJM* 281(23):1276–1285.

Figures 4-3a,b and 4-4: Eldh, P. and J. F. Silverman. 1974. Methods of studying the proximal left anterior descending coronary artery. *Radiology* 113(3):738–740. Copyright © 1974 by the Radiological Society of North America, Incorporated.

Figures 6-1 and 12-1: Killip, T., et al. Coronary artery surgery study. 1981. Part II. Published as a supplement to *Circulation* 63(6). American Heart Association Monograph No. 79. By permission of the American Heart Association, Inc.

Table 2-1: Modified from Conti, R. C. 1977. Reviews of contemporary laboratory methods: Coronary arteriography. *Circulation* 55(2):227–237.

Contents

Foreword

LEWIS WEXLER, M.D.

The difference between a skillful coronary angiographer and a plodder can be compared to the difference between a race car driver and a Sunday pleasure driver. The professional is in touch with the equipment, responding to variations in road conditions, the pitch of the motor, the pull on the wheel. But, more than the mechanics of driving, the real pro anticipates what will happen next and positions himself to take advantage of this knowledge.

A skillful angiographer also knows the equipment and has a feel for the way the catheter must be manipulated and the coronary vasculature displayed by proper table motion or image intensifier positioning. The mechanics of coronary arteriography can be learned easily, much like driving a car, but avoiding complications depends on anticipating them. Dr. Melvin P. Judkins has said that the most common complication of coronary angiography is an inadequate study. To avoid this complication, the professional angiographer applies a thorough understanding of three-dimensional coronary anatomy and the potential pathways of coronary collateral flow, an expectation of where disease will be located, an appreciation for the necessity of additional views to best display a particular anatomical segment, and the knowledge of how best to obtain that view. The expert can make these determinations almost instantly as the contrast filled vessels flash past on the video screen.

The skillful angiographer acquires this knowledge through assiduous application of the principles so lucidly enumerated in this text. Prior to the publication of this book by Dr. James F. Silverman, the fledgling angiographer lacked a simple, straightforward description of the foundations for successful performance and interpretation of coronary angiography. Indeed, it is an excellent review for any individual who is in training, or believes he has completed training, since it clearly emphasizes those aspects of arteriography that are often neglected in the trainee's desire to master the angiographic skills of catheter manipulation and contrast injection.

Dr. Silverman has received recognition as a dedicated teacher of coronary angiography. He has perfected the instructional techniques used in this book over more than a decade of teaching cardiology and radiology residents, fellows, and colleagues. These proven techniques are incorporated into the text, illustrations and, particularly, the model for transplanting the three-dimensional coronary anatomy into a two-dimensional ciné format. His unpretentious style of writing recognizes the needs of the novice, but is also filled with sufficient subtlety to benefit the experienced angiographer. Residents and fellows preparing for board examinations will find the text most useful, as have those who have attended the thorough board preparation courses offered by Dr. Silverman.

Dr. Wexler is the Professor of Radiology and Co-director of the Cardiac Catheterization Laboratory at Stanford University Medical Center.

Foreword

DONALD HARRISON, M.D.

Coronary Arteriography: An Introduction to Interpretation and Technique by Dr. James Silverman is an excellent introduction to the subject for those commencing fellowship training in cardiology and as a review for those more experienced in performing and interpreting coronary arteriograms. The straightforward discussion and description is clearly presented by someone who understands the need for this style of writing in medicine to clarify complex subjects.

The quality of the illustrations is excellent and provides an easy understanding for those uninitiated in the art of coronary arteriography. One of the excellent pieces of art work is the model of the heart, representing an easy way to interpret the distribution of the various vessels. This model allows the student to "three dimensionalize" vessel motion and eliminates much confusion when viewing arteriograms in the two-dimensional mode on a ciné projector. It also enhances understanding of angled views needed routinely for optimal vessel evaluation.

I think the text is a good one for the beginner in cardiology or radiology and represents the views of someone with great experience in performing coronary studies as well as someone who has made a career out of teaching using these methods.

I heartily endorse this book.

Dr. Harrison is the William G. Irwin Professor of Cardiology and Chief of the Cardiology Division at Stanford University School of Medicine.

Preface

As Alice walked down the road, she came to a fork. When she looked up, she saw a big Cheshire cat in one of the trees nearby.

"Would you tell me, please, which way I ought to go from here?"

"That depends a good deal on where you want to get to," said the Cat.

"I don't much care where—" said Alice.

"Then it doesn't matter which way you go," said the Cat.

Lewis Carroll
Alice in Wonderland

I try to remember that verse whenever I go to buy a new medical book. With the myriad titles, beautiful illustrations, and erudite explanations, I find it remarkably easy to forget "where I am going" in a bookstore. When my choice is between a basic text and a monograph, I seem to have a routine lapse of memory about what I really need to know. I have trouble admitting to myself that I may not remember, or may never have learned, anything about the subject I am now interested in. Therefore, although the basic text would be the obvious choice, I buy the advanced book instead—which teaches me some things, but always leaves me with that uncomfortable feeling that the basics are missing.

Coronary Angiography: An Introduction to Interpretation and Technique is a basic book. Although you can learn to read coronary arteriograms without it, you will, I assure you, have some trouble with the fundamentals of that skill. That is not because it is inherently too difficult, but is merely because available texts assume that you already know most of the basic material. The great radiologist, Evo Obrez, summarized the importance of basic principles with the statement, "you've got to put on your socks before your shoes." So it is, the basics before the advanced. The basics will not only teach you, but will provide the knowledge that will let you ask your own questions.

WHO IS THIS BOOK FOR?

Heart disease is the number one killer in the United States, and coronary artery disease is the major perpetrator. Anyone caring for cardiovascular patients will be involved with coronary artery disease, and inherent in that situation is the need to understand vascular studies necessary for diagnoses.

Coronary Angiography: An Introduction to Interpretation and Technique provides that information. Its purpose is to teach the reader about coronary angiography—not only how to look at arteriograms and interpret them, but to understand how and why such procedures are performed and how the results are reported and discussed.

The book will be useful for any physician or student who is interested in coronary angiography. It is not only suited for the reader who is merely interested in the subject, but also includes enough information to allow the cardiovascular surgeon to evaluate and decide if and where to operate.

Although this book starts at the beginning, it will be invaluable to those who are learning to perform this highly specialized procedure. This basic information is necessary for all radiologists and catheterization cardiologists, although both groups will ultimately know much more than this book has to offer by the end of their training.

The internist or general practitioner might also like to know just enough of the material to be involved in the decisions affecting their patients. One of the major objectives of the book is to provide such physicians with the terminology that will allow them to communicate with cardiac specialists.

THE HEART MODEL

Understanding coronary angiograms is really easy once you have overcome the major obstacle in learning to interpret them. The heart model included with this book is designed specifically to help you overcome that problem.

To the beginner viewing a coronary angiogram for the first time, the circulation appears as a complicated maze of vessels. In fact, the vessels are relatively few in number. What causes the confusion is the common perceptual problem that results when the three-dimensional heart is photographed on a two-dimensional plane. The posterior vessels are superimposed on the same surface as the anterior vessels, making them difficult to identify.

The problem is compounded by the positional change of each vessel as the heart is rotated for different angiographic views. To reach any useful understanding of coronary angiography, you must be able to identify the vessels in multiple views extending around the full axis of the heart. Until you understand the positional changes, you will make frequent errors in identifying vessels.

Use the model often as you go through the text. It will help you understand the special views, and will be particularly helpful in rotations through the axial planes. Ultimately, you will be able to understand the projections well enough to choose the appropriate views needed, should you be involved in doing or directing the study.

ACKNOWLEDGEMENTS

I would like to express my thanks to the people who helped a great deal in the production of this book.

1. To Lew Wexler and Diana Guthaner for their advice on the manuscript.
2. To Jeri Maislen for producing the manuscript and for her patience during the many revisions.
3. To Sue Harrington for her advice and understanding.
4. A special thanks to Bayard "Butch" Colyear from Stanford Instructional Media, who rendered the fine illustrations, particularly for his help in the model design.

James F. Silverman, M.D.

Assembling the Model

The heart model included in this book is designed specifically to help you understand how the cardiac vessels appear on an actual angiogram.

The model can be put together almost like a doll cutout, and when you have finished, you will have a very rough approximation of the heart with the major vessels drawn in their common positions. The model is printed on transparent plastic so that on rotating the model you can see through it to the vessels on the other side. With it, you can learn to recognize the vessels in any angiographic projection, including the special rotations such as the caudal and cranial views.

Take the model out of the book by carefully separating it from the base sheet along the perforated edges. Place the numbered tabs into the similarly numbered slots. The tabs are numbered in order for simple assembly, beginning with 0. *Note that each tab is cut along the bottom on each side. If you fold the sides of the tab back along the dotted lines before you push the tab through the corresponding slot, the tab edges will snap back and hold the tab in place.* (If you have real difficulties in manipulating the tabs, you can also tape the model together with transparent tape.) Be careful to orient the model so that you can read the names of the vessels—if you cannot, the model is inside out.

When the model is complete, it will have the semblance of a heart, slightly too shoe-shaped and flat-bottomed, but that allows the model to sit on a flat surface.

Here are a few points to remember as you use the model:

1. Although the base is flat and you will probably look at it as it sits in front of you, the heart is usually tipped apex down at about 15–20 degrees. The posterior vessels are really higher than the apex.

2. Tab No. 4 on the model is at the apex of the heart, where the anterior descending artery crosses from the anterior to the posterior surface. When Tab No. 4 is directly in front of you, the heart is in the left anterior oblique (LAO) position. Rotating the heart 30 degrees counterclockwise will put the heart in the anatomic position.

3. There are a number of routine projections obtained during angiographic filming. Starting at the anatomic position, routine projections are 60 degrees LAO, 45 degrees RAO (right anterior oblique), and lateral. These projections will be considered in detail in this book. When you use the model—and you should use it regularly throughout the first part of this book—you must be sure you can locate each vessel in each position.

So, put the heart model together, and let us begin.

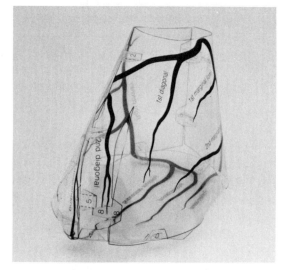

LAO

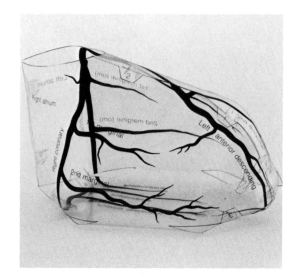

RAO

CHAPTER 1

Anatomy

You may think that a review of coronary anatomy is overly elementary in a book for practicing physicians. Surprisingly enough, it is not. In studying coronary angiograms, you will often view the heart in three dimensions and in a variety of projections. No matter how well you know chamber and vessel locations in one position, you will find that movement of these structures during rotation will make them difficult to recognize at first. Therefore, if you are to understand coronary angiography, you must have a solid understanding of coronary anatomy. Hence, a review.

SURFACE AND CHAMBER ANATOMY

Figure 1-1 shows (a) anterior, (b) lateral, (c) left anterior oblique (LAO), and (d) right anterior oblique (RAO) views of the heart. The important structures to note are:

1. Superior vena cava (SVC)
2. Right atrium
3. Inferior vena cava (IVC)
4. Aorta
5. Pulmonary artery
6. Right ventricle
7. Pulmonary veins
8. Left atrium
9. Left ventricle
10. Right coronary artery (RCA)
11. Left anterior descending artery (LAD)
12. Left circumflex artery (CIRC)
13. Coronary sinus

Remember, the heart is rotated during coronary filming. You must get a sense of the anterior–posterior (three-dimensional) location of all the cardiac structures. Very anterior structures, such as the left anterior descending artery (LAD) and the pulmonary artery, or posterior structures, such as the circumflex artery and coronary sinus, move a great deal during filming with even slight rotations of the heart. The structures on the lateral aspect of the heart (marginal and diagonal branches), however, will move much less during similar rotations. It is not necessary to dwell on surface anatomy; it is the spatial location of structures that you must remember.

FIGURE 1-1.

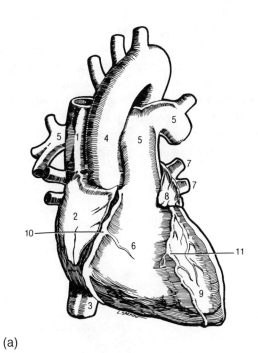

(a)

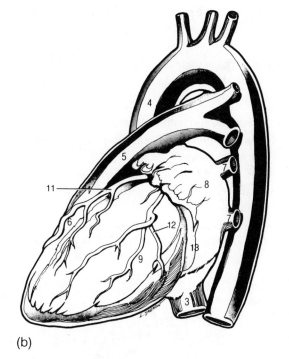

(b)

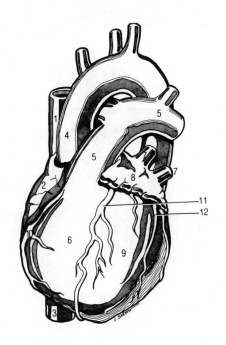

(c)

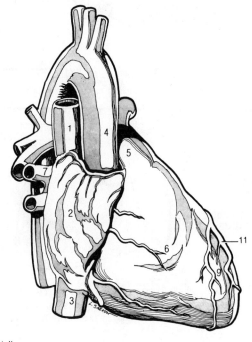

(d)

Figure 1-2 illustrates chamber and valve anatomy. (Note: the structures shaded in the drawings carry oxygenated blood, and the unshaded structures carry venous return.) Important points to remember about chamber and valve anatomy are that:

- The aortic and mitral valves are contiguous.
- The pulmonary valve is anterior and higher than the aortic valve.
- The tricuspid and pulmonary valves are separated by the pulmonary conus (infundibulum).
- The left ventricle is ellipsoid and posterior.
- The right ventricle is trapezoidal and anterior.

When we perform a ventriculogram during coronary arteriography, we will study the left ventricle. We will be able to evaluate wall thickness, chamber volume, ejection fraction, contractility, and valve motion. Thus, ventriculography will allow a really functional evaluation of the heart before surgery. This evaluation, as you will see, may be the most valuable prognostic sign about operability or about longevity after surgery.

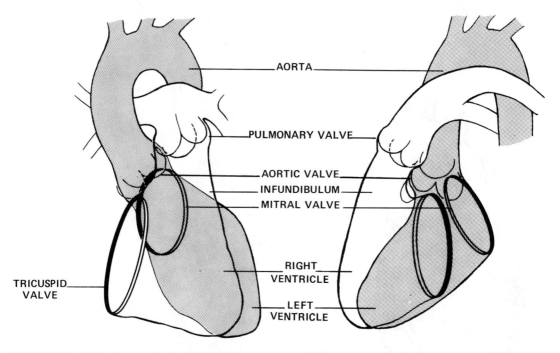

FIGURE 1-2. Stippled portion in each projection carries oxygenated blood—mitral valve, left ventricle, aortic valve, aorta. Clear portion in each projection carries venous return—tricuspid valve, right ventricle, pulmonary valve, pulmonary artery.

CORONARY ARTERIOGRAPHIC ANATOMY

Circle and Loop Method

In 1970, Dr. Marvin Davis developed a simple but instructive method, the circle and loop method, to help explain coronary arteriographic anatomy. I would like you to use this system to solidify your understanding of vessel location and nomenclature. Get the circle and loop approach down pat. If you can identify the four main vessels forming the circle and loop, you will be able to identify all the other vessels as well. More important, this system will help you understand the vessel location in various projections.

In Figure 1-3, the anteroposterior (AP) and posteroanterior (PA) anatomic structures are paired with a drawing to illustrate the circle and loop method. Four branches make up the circle and loop. For the circle, they are the right coronary artery and the circumflex coronary artery. The loop is made up of the left anterior descending and posterior descending arteries. Note the location of those four major coronary branches on the model and on the anatomic drawing. Remember as you study the circle and loop method that:

- Coronary arteriography allows multiple views of the vessels.
- The difficulty for most viewers is to understand the movement of the vessels from view to view.
- You should note the location of each vessel, thinking three-dimensionally, as we move from projection to projection.

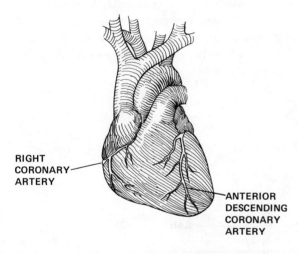

RIGHT CORONARY ARTERY

ANTERIOR DESCENDING CORONARY ARTERY

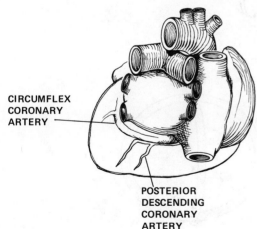

CIRCUMFLEX CORONARY ARTERY

POSTERIOR DESCENDING CORONARY ARTERY

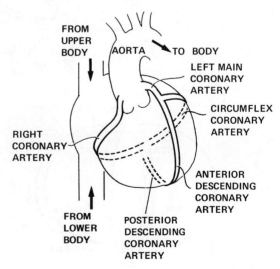

FROM UPPER BODY

AORTA

TO BODY

LEFT MAIN CORONARY ARTERY

CIRCUMFLEX CORONARY ARTERY

RIGHT CORONARY ARTERY

ANTERIOR DESCENDING CORONARY ARTERY

FROM LOWER BODY

POSTERIOR DESCENDING CORONARY ARTERY

FIGURE 1-3.

In the circle and loop method, there are two planes, the atrioventricular groove (AV) (stippled) and the interventricular septum (IV) (cross-hatched), wherein reside the major vessels (Figure 1-4a). In the AV groove lie the right coronary artery (RCA) and the circumflex branch (CIRC) of the left coronary artery. These vessels make up the circle of the circle and loop. In the IV septum are the anterior descending branch of the left coronary artery (LAD) and the posterior descending branch (PDA), which can come from either the right or left coronary artery. These two branches form the loop. Note the orientation of the circle and loop in the upper graphic presentation in the AP projection. Figure 1-4b and c also show the relationship of the AV and IV grooves but are drawn in the standard right anterior oblique (RAO) and left anterior oblique (LAO) projections.

Figure 1-5 gives another, slightly less diagrammatic, view of the location of the vessels in the AV and IV planes in the RAO and LAO projections. Remember that in the circle and loop approach, the circle is on the AV groove, which separates the atria from the ventricles. The loop is in the interventricular septum and separates the right from the left ventricle.

Now, if you think that you know these vessels, go to Figure 1-6 and label the major vessels *and* heart chambers in the drawing. Note again that in the RAO view, everything to the left of the AV groove is atrium; vessels going in that direction, whether from the right or left coronary artery, are atrial vessels.

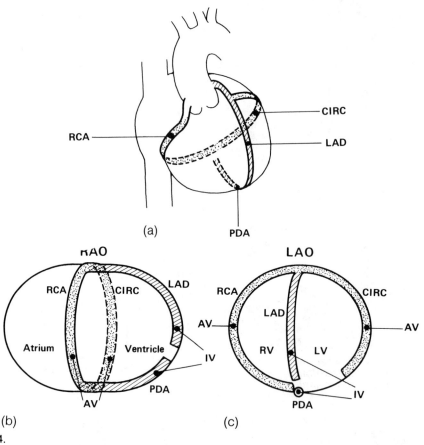

FIGURE 1-4.

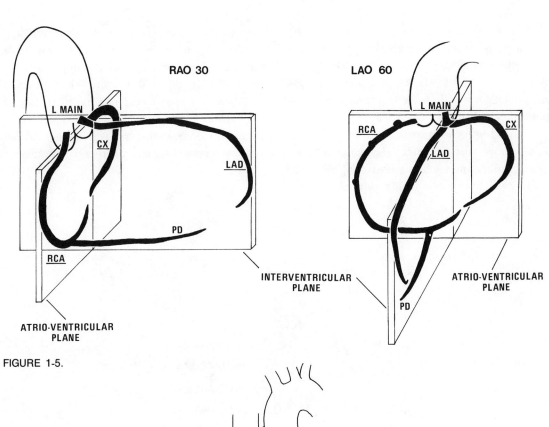

RAO 30

LAO 60

L MAIN

CX

LAD

PD

RCA

ATRIO-VENTRICULAR
PLANE

INTERVENTRICULAR
PLANE

L MAIN

RCA

CX

LAD

PD

ATRIO-VENTRICULAR
PLANE

FIGURE 1-5.

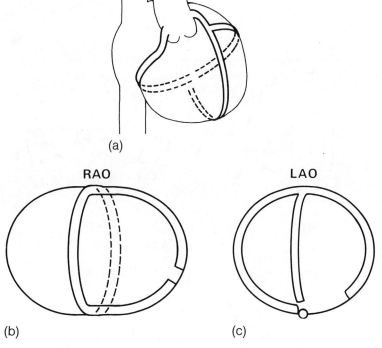

(a)

RAO

LAO

FIGURE 1-6.   (b)   (c)

The next step is to learn the remaining important coronary artery branches (Figure 1-7). Although the terminology for these branches varies from author to author, the simplest and most descriptive language is the most appropriate for communication with another physician.

Note that branches emanating from vessels in the AV groove, that is, from the right coronary and left circumflex arteries, are vessels that emanate from around the *margin* of the ventricle. These vessels are appropriately called *marginals*, whether they originate from the right coronary or left circumflex coronary artery. They are numbered (1), (2), (3), and so on. (The left-sided marginals are often called oblique marginals or OM-branches and the right-sided marginals acute marginals.) Branches that come off of the LAD, you will note, course *diagonally* across the ventricular

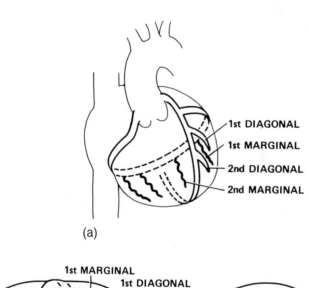

(a)

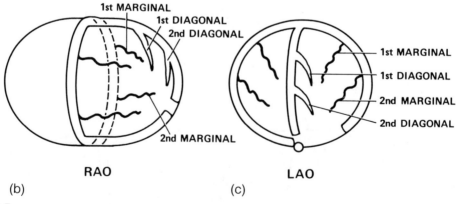

RAO

(b)

LAO

(c)

FIGURE 1-7.

surface. These branches are called *diagonals* and are numbered in order as they come off from the major trunk. Figure 1-8 shows the additional vessels as they relate to the "planar" localization.

We have now considered the location and nomenclature of eight vessels—four major vessels (LAD, PDA, CIRC, and RCA) and four minor vessels (first and second marginals and first and second diagonals). It is important to realize that most surgery on the heart is performed on these vessels.

The common denominators are vessel size and the amount of myocardium perfused. These vessels are usually larger than 1 mm and thus are amenable to bypass surgery. Therefore, knowing these eight vessels will allow you to evaluate the coronary anatomy and assess the degree of surgically reparable disease.

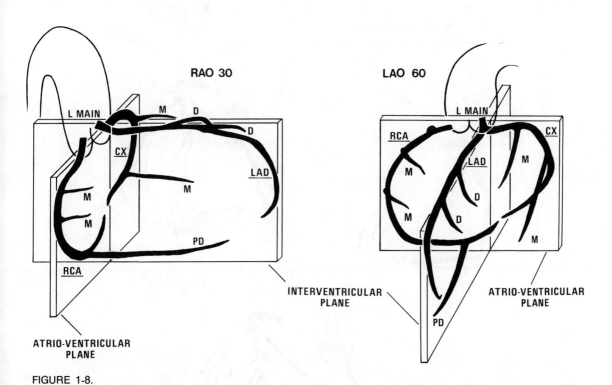

FIGURE 1-8.

Applying the Circle and Loop Method

The next step is to relate the circle and loop configuration to real vessels. Figure 1-9 shows an LAO grouping with a graphic circle and loop at the top compared to a true angiographic composite at the bottom. The right coronary injection is to the left in the middle, and the left coronary injection is to the right. This figure should convince you that the circle and loop configuration is fairly valid. Can you identify the PDA, right marginals, diagonals, left marginals, and left main coronary artery in the composite? Some are easy to identify, and some are hard because of the overlap of vessels. For this reason, multiple projections are necessary.

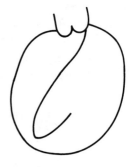

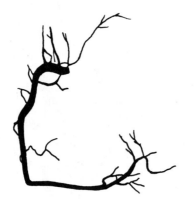 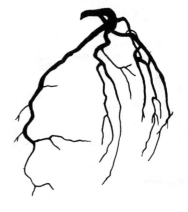

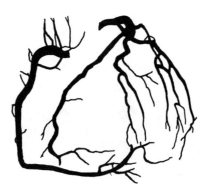

FIGURE 1-9.

Figure 1-10 shows the RAO projection with a similar group of pictures. Again, note the circle and loop representation in the final angiographic composite. In this projection the PDA and left marginals are easier to identify; however, even though there are only eight or so important vessels, the presence of many smaller vessels makes their evaluation difficult. Later in this text we will discuss how vessel movement during cineangiographic (ciné) filming will help you identify the important vessels.

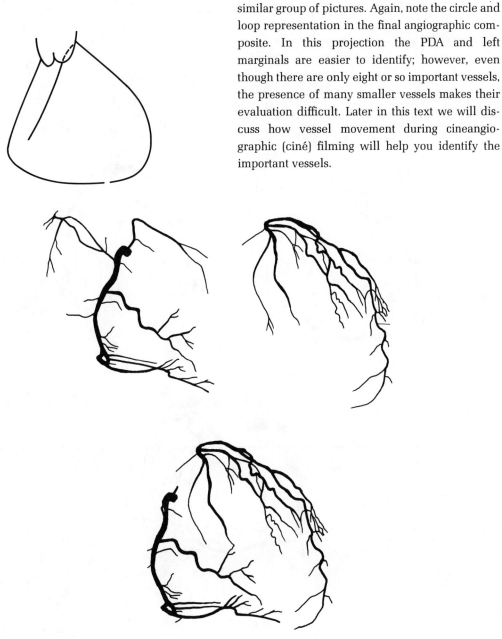

FIGURE 1-10.

As a final review, use both the LAO and RAO composites (Figures 1-11 and 1-12) to see if you can identify all of the branches in one view before and after they are rotated into the other projection. The vessels in the LAO are numbered. Try naming them and matching them up with the appropriately lettered vessel in the RAO. (The answers are on page 14.)

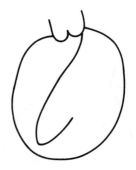

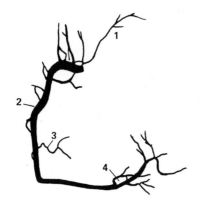

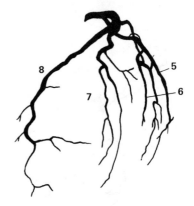

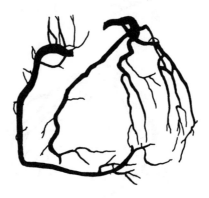

FIGURE 1-11.

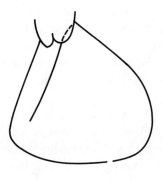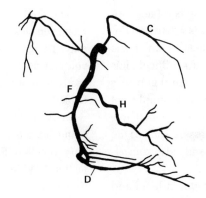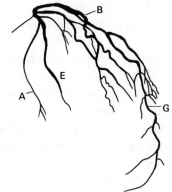

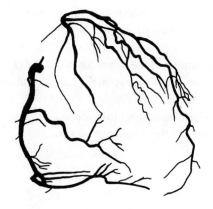

FIGURE 1-12.

LAO**
Name of Vessel

RAO
Letter Representing
Same Vessel in RAO

1. _____   _____
2. _____   _____
3. _____   _____
4. _____   _____
5. _____   _____
6. _____   _____
7. _____   _____
8. _____   _____

CORONARY ARTERIOGRAPHIC ANATOMY

In this exercise, the vessels have rotated approximately 90 degrees (the LAO is rotated 60 degrees and the RAO 35–45 degrees in these projections). If you found the exercise difficult, it is probably because of the very problem this book's heart model is designed to help: It is simply not easy to visualize a three-dimensional object that is being rotated. A few additional vessels, such as the conus artery (an important collateral), also complicate matters.

Before moving on, take the model in hand and hold it in an AP projection. The overlap of vessels explains why this view is not routinely obtained; however, note how visualization of certain vessels is enhanced in various degrees of RAO and LAO rotation. For example, observe how difficult it is to see the beginning of the diagonals in the RAO but how well they are then seen in the LAO. Similarly, the PDA is difficult to define in the LAO projection because it "comes right at" the viewer. In the RAO, the full length of this vessel can be seen.

The final graphic-arteriographic constructs will move you closer to reality—that is, angiographic reality. The graphics are copies of the angiograms. If you can identify all the vessels you see, you are ready to move out of the anatomy section of this book.

Look at the LAO pairs in Figure 1-13. Name the major branches as you move down the right coronary injection (Figure 1-13a). Now go to the left injection (Figure 1-13b). Make the circle and loop. Can you name the vessels? Do you know which surfaces they are on—anterior or posterior? If you can do that, go to the RAO set in Figure 1-14.

KEY	ANSWER
1. Conus	C
2. RCA	F
3. 2nd Marg.	H
4. PDA	D
5. 2nd OM	E
6. CX	A
7. DIAG	B
8. LAD	G

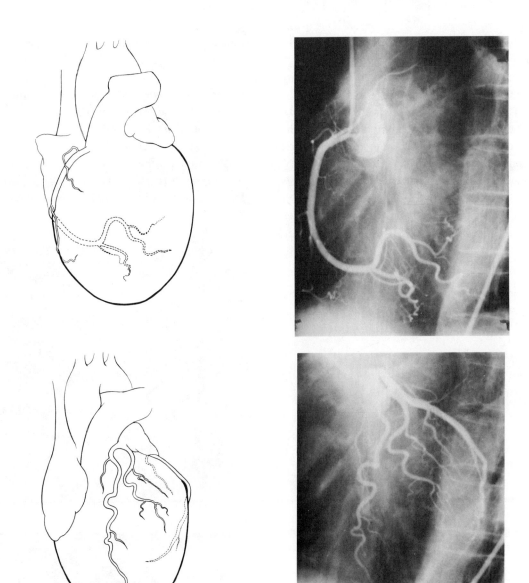

(a)

(b)

FIGURE 1-13.

In Figure 1-14a and b, the RAO set, move down the right coronary artery. Can you name the branches? Do you see the atrial branches? Where is the posterior descending artery?

Go to the left injection (Figure 1-14b). Do you see the catheter? Can you identify the vessels? Where are the left main coronary artery, the LAD, the diagonal branches, and the first marginal? Do you know which surface the vessels are on?

Before leaving the RAO, notice that some vessels appear to cross others. How can that be? Re-member, coronary vessels do not cross. If they appear to cross in angiography, it is because they are on different portions of a wall arc, and rotary wall motion moves one segment in one direction and the other segment in another, giving the sem-blance of crossing. In reality, they are separated spatially. We will discuss this further in Chapter 7.

We are ready to move on to the next portion of this primer. It is crucial that you have a good feel for vessel locations in different degrees of rotation. If not, review this section before going on.

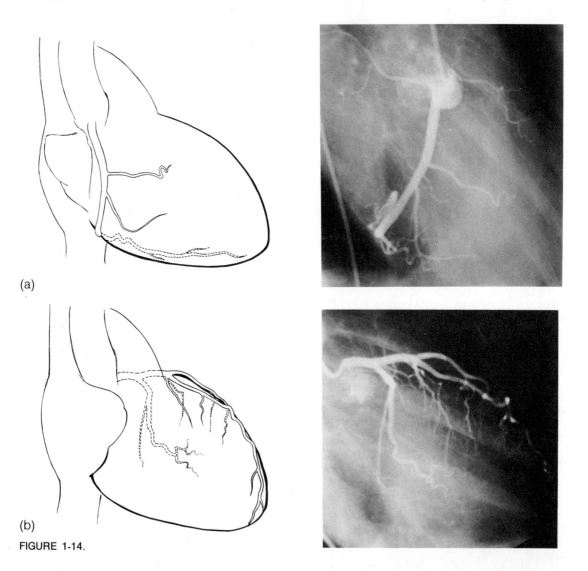

(a)

(b)

FIGURE 1-14.

CHAPTER 2

Indications for Coronary Arteriography

It was well stated by Gensini that "the primary goal of coronary arteriography is the identification, localization, and assessment of obstructive lesions present within the arteries of the heart." From Gensini's statement, I assume that the information so gathered would be used in a meaningful way, leading to surgical, medical, or, perhaps, no therapy for the patient. As the years have passed and arteriography has become very safe, though the goal has remained the same as stated, the population that has undergone this procedure at our institution has changed markedly.

SYMPTOMATIC PATIENTS

Ten years ago, patient selection was clearly affected by the gravity of the procedure, and those studied were mainly symptomatic with acute or chronic anginal syndromes. Those patients were essentially evaluated for surgery (though the surgical techniques, results, and indications were in their early stages at that time). As the years have passed, coronary arteriography has become routine and safe, as has coronary artery surgery (coronary artery bypass surgery is the second most common operation at Stanford University

Hospital). Also, studies have appeared that suggest some patients not only have relief of pain following surgery but live longer. This finding, along with the low risks involved in coronary arteriography, has encouraged the performance of such studies by even conservative physicians, who in the past might have treated patients with angina without performing an angiographic study. Physicians can find security in knowing their patients do not need surgery from a length-of-survival point of view. Therefore, an increasing number of patients with acute or chronic ischemic symptoms are now undergoing study. They are the group most often studied.

As arteriography has become safer and increasingly available, more and more patients with chest pain from unknown causes are being studied, in addition to patients with valid ischemic symptoms. These are patients with unusual chest pain syndromes, in whom knowledge of the presence or absence of coronary artery disease would be critical to patient management. There are numerous patients of this sort, and they are as frustrating to the cardiologist as patients with ill-defined low back pain are to the orthopedist or those with peculiar headaches are to the neurologist. Each of these physician groups tries its best medically or psychologically but often is forced to use definitive tests to help manage patients. Therefore, patients having chest pain of unknown causes are another group indicated for study.

After some thought, you might realize that because the chest pain is unusual and because coronary artery lesions may not have reached a symptomatic stage, finding disease in this group of patients might not have anything to do with the chest pain! Then what do you do? Sometimes, diagnostic examinations create more problems than they solve.

ASYMPTOMATIC PATIENTS

Many of the patients studied (again because of two factors—safety of the procedure and data that cardiovascular surgery may prolong life) are those with abnormal results from noninvasive tests such as a stress electrocardiogram or an isotope study (thallium or other isotopes, depending on the institution) that evaluates myocardial blood flow. Along with many preventive health measures now thought important, and most particularly for certain age groups, noninvasive tests of cardiac function have become a common part of many yearly physical examinations. Needless to say, because these studies are done on many sedentary individuals, real disease is sometimes uncovered and further angiographic study may be indicated. However, because these noninvasive studies have problems with both sensitivity and specificity, a group of patients may become candidates for arteriography when it may not be indicated.

There may be other indications for study, depending on the physician or the institution. A good example, which varies among physicians, is the study of patients undergoing valve surgery. In aortic valve disease, the patient population is old, and sometimes there is significant coronary artery disease that has been asymptomatic because the valve disease has determined the degree of patient activity and thus inhibited the appearance of angina symptoms. These patients are studied routinely in some institutions.

The foregoing is only a short list, of course, of indications for coronary arteriography. Table 2-1 is a short summary of indications, including a few that have not been discussed in the text. The list can be lengthened or shortened by your experiences or practices. What I have presented in this chapter is a realistic starting point.

TABLE 2-1   Indications for Coronary Arteriography

Symptomatic Patients
Acute anginal syndromes
Chronic anginal syndromes
Chest pain of unknown etiology
Asymptomatic Patients
Positive stress ECG or abnormal isotope study
Before valvular surgery
Postoperative evaluation of surgery
Myocardiopathy evaluation
Unusual Indications
Vessel location in congenital heart disease
Definition of vessel abnormalities such as fistulas, aneurysms, traumatic injuries

CHAPTER 3

Foundations for Vessel Evaluation

To obtain diagnostic arteriograms, it is critical to obtain films in proper projections and with adequate injections. We will discuss these subjects in upcoming chapters.

At this point, however, you must be introduced to some material that is not exactly basic but that is nonetheless crucial for explaining, prognosticating, and converting angiographic data into a diagnostic opinion. To be able to do this you need to know some of the language of coronary arteriography. I think you will find that recognition of these issues now will make later information more meaningful and easier to understand and remember.

VESSEL DESCRIPTIONS

The first area to consider is what coronary arteries look like. Although the main cause of coronary artery abnormalities is atherosclerotic vascular disease, the presentation of such abnormalities can differ greatly. It is important to understand such differences and the flow dynamics that follow in coronary arterial evaluation. The description of the various changes is also important; the vessel description becomes part of the report, which must use terminology that is universally understood. Figure 3-1 shows some of the many coronary arterial changes. A variety of methods are used to describe vessel abnormalities. The important thing, though, is to use names that have similar meanings to various film readers, because a report is often all that is available for decision making. Thus, the nomenclature needs to be descriptive but concise, which can be difficult for several reasons. First, in a single vessel, multiple types of lesions may flow together.

Second, and more important, there are no finite definitions for all the abnormalities. Thus, one name tends to merge into another. Some general terms that follow apply to the examples in Figure 3-1.

1. *Normal.* Smooth walls; gradual tapering
2. *Discrete Lesion.* Well-defined narrowing less than 0.5 cm; adjacent vessel relatively normal
3. *Multiple Discrete Lesions.* Several narrowings less than 0.5 cm; separated by relatively normal vessel
4. *Discrete Aneurysmal Lesion.* Dilated segment that is larger than normal; may be preceded by normal or abnormal vessel
5. *Multiple Aneurysmal Lesions.* Dilated segments that are larger than normal
6. *Diffuse Disease.* Long segments of abnormal vessels without interposed normal vessel
7. *Tubular.* Well-defined narrowing greater than 1 cm in length

It won't be long before you begin to differ with others in describing lesions. Most of it is really semantics and, in terms of patient evaluation for surgery, degrees of narrowing will be more important. At this point, however, it is useful for you to appreciate the variety of disease forms that are bunched under the terminology "coronary artery disease."

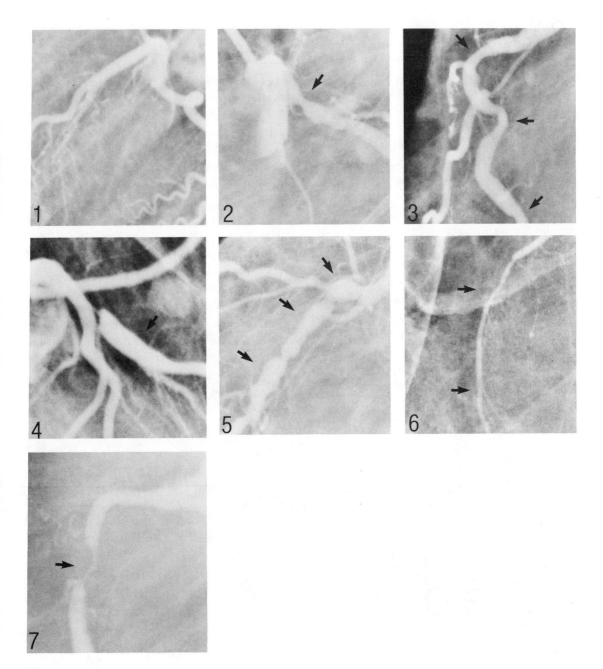

FIGURE 3-1.

DOMINANCE

Dominance refers to the blood supply to the inferior wall of the left ventricle. To understand the discussion of dominance you must be familiar with two vessels not yet introduced—the posterolateral branches. The nomenclature for these branches describes their location on the left ventricular wall. The main branch in this area is, of course, the posterior descending artery. Whether it is from the right or left coronary arterial system, its location is usually on the intraventricular septum. The two new branches are numbered from the posterior descending artery as the first and second posterolateral branches. Occasionally, there is a third or even a fourth posterolateral branch.

As mentioned, dominance (dominant coronary circulation) refers to the coronary arterial blood supply to the posteroinferior wall of the left ventricle. Dominance has nothing to do with the *predominant* blood supply—that is, which vessel supplies most of the blood to the ventricle. That vessel is essentially always the left coronary artery, because the left coronary artery supplies the bulk

of the intraventricular septum, as well as a large portion of the left ventricular free wall. Instead, dominance merely defines the anatomic configurations of the vessels to the posteroinferior left ventricle. (Little will be said of the right ventricle in these discussions. Most coronary artery disease that you will study will involve decisions about the left ventricular blood supply.)

The possible configurations for dominance are three: Dominance can be left, right, or balanced. These are best understood in the LAO projection (Figure 3-2). In right dominance the right coronary artery gives off the posterior descending artery and the major posterolateral branches. In left dominance the circumflex artery gives off the posterolateral branches and terminates giving off the posterior descending artery. In the balanced configuration, the posterior descending artery is from the right coronary artery and the posterolateral branches are from the left coronary artery.

The importance of dominance relates mainly to the hazards of coronary artery disease. If an individual is left dominant (Figure 3-2b), the entire left

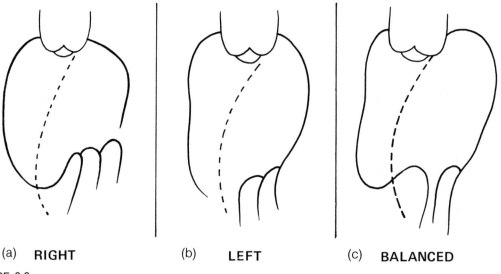

(a) **RIGHT**   (b) **LEFT**   (c) **BALANCED**

FIGURE 3-2.

ventricular blood supply is controlled by the patency of the left main coronary artery (thus the hazard of a lesion in that area). In addition, the right coronary artery is a small vessel in that configuration, so there is no good-sized potential collateral. Therefore, if you had your choice, you would want right dominant or balanced circulation, because you could lose one vessel and still have a portion of the left ventricular blood supply available and a good potential collateral in place.

LEFT MAIN CORONARY ARTERY DISEASE AND EQUIVALENTS

Because we have discussed dominance and the effect of dominance on coronary disease evaluation, this is an appropriate time to discuss left main coronary artery disease. Although we have been doing coronary arteriography for more than ten years, only during the last few years have data appeared to support the concept that certain types of lesions require surgery. "Require" means more than symptom alleviation. It means preventing sudden death or increasing life span.

The first such lesion identified was a left main coronary artery lesion (Figure 3-3a). This lesion is morbid in any type of dominance but is catastrophic with left dominant circulation. You should understand this because in a left dominant heart, an obstruction of the left main coronary artery would leave the left ventricle with virtually no blood supply. The right coronary artery is usually small in this configuration and is therefore a poor supplier of collaterals. Thus, sudden closure of this left main coronary artery is often fatal.

An "equivalent" to a left main coronary lesion in the left dominant circulation is a right dominant circulation with both left main and right main coronary lesions (Figure 3-3b). Another example might be a proximal right, proximal LAD, and proximal circumflex in the anatomy shown in Figure 3-2b. These are equivalents in theory but obviously are not exactly the same as left dominance with a left main lesion. Although the other combinations could be as serious, it is very unlikely that two or three high-grade lesions would close simultaneously. However, with high-grade lesions in the alternative areas, the same caution is often taken by cardiologists and surgeons, and such arteriographic findings are soon followed by surgery.

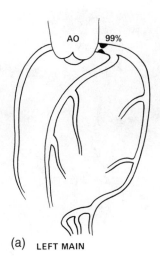

(a) LEFT MAIN

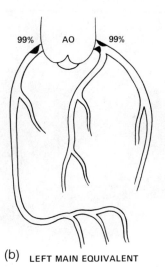

(b) LEFT MAIN EQUIVALENT

FIGURE 3-3.

EVALUATION OF VESSEL NARROWINGS

A careful assessment of the degree of vessel narrowing is a critical part of coronary arteriographic evaluation.

Obtaining Accurate Angiographic Data

Certain rules must be followed to ensure that the angiograms will give you adequate information on which to base your evaluation. First, the lumen must be clearly visualized to allow you to measure the vessels. This requires a firm hand injection. Second, vessels can only be evaluated when the margins are well defined with radiopaque contrast. If you are going to measure vessel diameters, the lumen should be clearly visualized and the wall margins must be well defined with radiopaque contrast. This requires a firm hand injection and an injection speed of at least 3 mL/sec for 2 sec.

Multiple Views. Most important, you must see multiple views to be sure of your evaluation. Remember, the evaluation from the view in which the vessel appears narrowest is usually the correct one.

A vessel is a circular tube, and no matter how you rotate it you cannot make the normal dimensions look abnormally small.

You can, however, be fooled by vessel overlap (Figure 3-4), which makes the vessel appear large. You then may be fooled because the adjoining segment looks abnormally small.

In Figure 3-4a, a conglomeration of multiple vessels (arrows) appears to be one very large trunk. If the LAD (a) is compared to this trunk, it will "measure" narrowed. Figure 3-4b demonstrates that, in reality, all the vessels taper fairly normally. Note how much of the proximal LAD (a), diagonal (b), and circumflex (c) was hidden in the conglomeration of proximal vessels. This is a common problem when viewing the LAD in the LAO projection, in which the proximal vessels superimpose upon each other, making the proximal left coronary artery branches so large. As the left anterior descending artery begins to descend in the interventricular groove, it looks abnormally small compared to these proximal overlapped segments. This is a common error made by novices to coronary arteriography. Experience—and a check of other views to confirm normality—will minimize such mistakes.

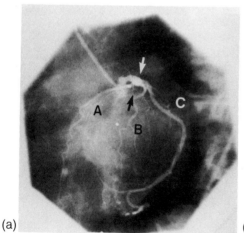

(a)

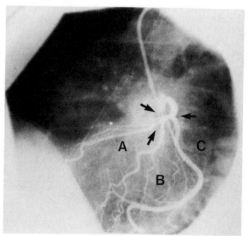

(b)

FIGURE 3-4.

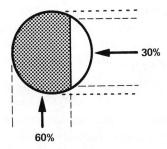

30%

60%

FIGURE 3-5.

Measurement of Symmetric and Eccentric Lesions

Lesions are measured a variety of ways. You can use a ruler or calipers to measure the vessel on the projector screen, or the image can be projected onto a suitable wall or screen to magnify the vessel. As long as the edges remain sharp, the more you magnify the vessel, the more accurate your measurement will be. In most centers, narrowings are described as a percent decrease in the cross-sectional luminal diameter compared to a normal segment. For example, a 50% lesion means that the cross-sectional measurement was half that of the adjacent normal segment. The calculation does not measure area loss. If you wish to convert to an area measurement, simply use the formula $A = \pi r^2$. But remember, almost everyone uses cross-sectional diameter, and even if an area measurement seems more accurate, you are communicating to others and the information has to be understood. If you plan to use an area measurement, make a special note to let others know.

Another reason multiple views must be obtained is that lesions may be eccentric. A vessel such as the one shown in the cross section in Figure 3-5, when viewed from one direction, might appear only mildly abnormal, with a narrowing of 30%. When viewed from another angle, the vessel will be shown to have the much more significant narrowing of 60%. There is one good sign that suggests that a lesion may be eccentric and more significant than it appears. When you view a vessel along its length, if the density (whiteness) of one segment appears to be less than that of a neighboring portion, this observation suggests that other views will show the lesion in its true dimension. Be aware, however, that muscular pressure on the vessel or pulsatile blood flow can also create such density changes.

Note the following diagrams. Figure 3-6a shows an eccentric narrowing, Figure 3-6b a symmetric lesion. Both are 50% narrowings if we compare the lesion to the proximal segment. But for Figure 3-6a, the area calculation will be:

$$A = \pi r^2$$
$$A = 3.1 \times 4^2$$
$$A = 49.6 \text{ mm}$$
$$50\% \text{ eccentric} = 24.8 \text{ mm remaining}$$
$$= 50\% \text{ area gone}$$

For Figure 3-6b, the area measure will be:

$$A = \pi r^2$$
$$A = 3.1 \times 2^2$$
$$A = 12.4 \text{ mm}$$
$$50\% \text{ symmetric} = 12.44 \text{ mm remaining}$$
$$= 75\% \text{ area gone}$$

Thus, the symmetric 50% narrowing should carry a different weight in your mind than a 50% eccentric lesion. The area loss is clearly different. Unfortunately, area is not used to any extent in the lan-guage between angiographers. But you should remember the concept when evaluating vessels.

The problems with measurements of any kind (calipers, rulers) are that:

- Sometimes no nearly normal segment is nearby—often none exist—for comparison. If the whole vessel is somewhat narrowed, you can only guess at what percentage to use.
- The vessel wall edges may be indistinct. Whether this is film technique or inadequate contrast, the result is that accuracy is lost.
- The vessel may be too small for any accuracy regardless of how it is measured. Vessels smaller than 1 mm are difficult with either ruler or calipers.

Location, Numbers, and Lengths of Lesions

Location. In most patients, coronary artery disease affects the first 5 cm of the major vessels. It is also critical to remember that routine coronary ar-

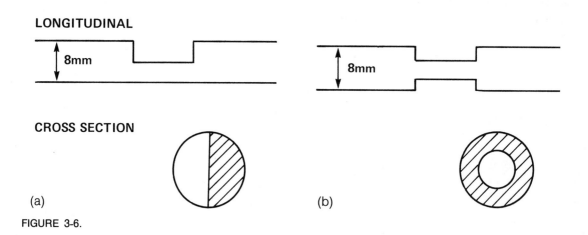

LONGITUDINAL

8mm

8mm

CROSS SECTION

(a)

(b)

FIGURE 3-6.

tery disease does not affect intramyocardial coronary arteries. Therefore, what you see in the surface vessels is essentially the extent of the disease. This fact, along with the proximal location of the lesions, is why bypass vein grafting has been so successful. It essentially creates a new, normal conduit to the remainder of the circulation. The diseased part is bypassed.

Number. The number of lesions is important, since a successful bypass must extend beyond the most severe lesion if surgery is to be beneficial. The procedure need not bypass all lesions, but downstream disease cannot be high grade or flow to the myocardium will remain diminished. Surgery fails for several reasons. First, as mentioned, if a distal lesion is missed and not bypassed, there continues to be diminished flow to the ischemic area. Second, if flow down the graft is inadequate for any reason, the graft often closes. Note that if the proximal portion of the bypassed vessel has also closed, which is often the case after a graft is placed, the patient is left with less blood flow than he or she had before surgery!

Length. Length of lesion is important and should be part of your evaluation. Although usually not measured and calculated, long lesions are more significant than short ones. Therefore, in evaluating the coronary arteries, length as well as the percentage of narrowing must be considered.

Significance

The question of significance will probably be raised during your first coronary artery review session. Suppose you think the LAD is 60% narrowed. Is it a significant narrowing?

The term *significance* implies that a narrowing is of high enough grade to prevent, under a variety of circumstances, an adequate blood supply from reaching the area of myocardium supplied by the vessel. Definite evidence of significant narrowing is collateral flow to the vessel distal to its lesion. Less definitive evidence is slowed flow in a vessel compared to its neighbor.

But remember, as you are evaluating narrowings and trying to decide their significance, you are looking at the vessel at rest. A graph of blood flow versus narrowing percentage at rest and during exercise looks something like that in Figure 3-7. Looking at the graph, you can see that, at rest, a vessel needs to be approximately 80% narrowed before flow begins to diminish. This implies that a vessel needs to be 80% narrowed for a lesion to be

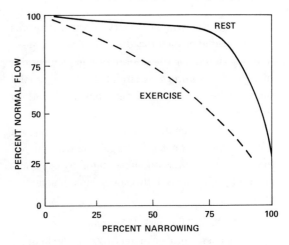

FIGURE 3-7. At rest, flow falls off at 80% narrowing, with exercise, at 50%–60%.

significant. However, the exercise line shows that when vessels are 50%–60% narrowed, flow falls to below half of normal. Because anginal pain usually occurs with exertion, it is assumed that when a lesion is about 50%–60% of the normal cross-sectional diameter, the lesion is significant. Consider the subtlety of your diagnostic opinion when there is a 50% symmetric, long (greater than 1 cm) lesion versus a 50% eccentric, short lesion. You will need to translate these variables into a conclusion that indicates whether a lesion is significant, that is, whether it has caused myocardial flow to decrease. These are the nuances of diagnostic evaluation. The best evaluation will be one that uses every shred of angiographic information and correlates it with clinical findings and other laboratory results. Angiographic diagnosis is clearly not an exact science, but the more you know and the more rational your thinking, the better an angiographer you will be.

ANGIOGRAPHIC VS SURGICAL OR PATHOLOGIC EVALUATION

Many years ago, when coronary arteriography was a budding diagnostic procedure, the obvious question was raised: Do the arteriographic pictures depict in vivo findings accurately? It is a crucial question, because surgical decisions are based on this relationship.

Interestingly enough, the answer depends on who you ask. If you ask a surgeon, he will tell you that lesions are often underestimated by using angiography. He comes to this conclusion in a variety of ways:

1. He "feels" the vessel at surgery.
2. He passes probes of varying sizes up to or beyond the lesion.
3. He observes color or motion of the myocardium after a bypass.
4. He measures flow before and after bypass.

I have worked with surgeons who have used all of these methods. In my experience, the angiographic picture is more accurate compared to Methods 1 and 2. The surgeon obviously cannot "feel" degrees of narrowing, and the probe technique is less valuable because it is performed on the nonbeating, undistended heart with nondistended vessels. I suspect some vessels are needlessly bypassed because of this reasoning. Therefore, I try to persuade these surgeons to depend on arteriograms.

For those who declare motion improvement of the ventricle to support their claims, I request before-surgery and after-surgery ventriculograms, which can provide concrete evidence that a change occurred after bypass. Unfortunately, invasive methods are not popular in the postoperative period. Those surgeons using Method 4 should send you back for another look at your study.

If a pathologist tells you that you were wrong, you should again inquire about his method:

1. He may merely cut across a diseased vessel during postmortem examination.
2. He may fill the vessel with barium solution and take a radiograph.
3. He may fill the vessel with a gel that solidifies into a cast.

Method 1 is fraught with error because there is no distention of the vessel, and the prediction is based on non-fluid-filled lumen. Even though the vessel walls may be thick or calcified, they are often very distensible. Thus, comparing the empty postmortem vessel to the contrast-filled antemortem vessel is not reasonable.

Method 2 or 3, filling with barium or cast material, necessitates tying off all tributaries and injecting them at the same pressure as the patient's systolic pressure to reach a comparable dimension. Pathology studies using these methods have supported the accuracy of angiographic diagnosis or have suggested errors on angiography. These studies raise some question about the dynamics of the vessel wall in the autopsy room. Therefore, you may have significant reservations when a pathologist tells you that you have underestimated the lesion.

Another important discrepancy became apparent when pathologists found coronary artery disease in two special groups of patients who historically or during prior angiographic studies appeared to be normal. The first group found to have such coronary artery disease was very young war casualties. The other group is the small number of patients who die of cardiac or noncardiac causes who have had normal coronaries on prior coronary arteriography.

Although these occurrences may seem paradoxical, there is a reasonable explanation. Remember, the roentgenogram shows only the lumen and not the vessel wall. The angiographer will know that the vessel is narrowed only when a diseased segment is narrower in comparison to a healthier segment of the same vessel. Take a look at Figure 3-8. To an angiographer, both of the lumens may appear equally normal: Figure 3-8b could be called abnormal only in comparison to another truly normal segment close by. When we say that a vessel is angiographically normal, the lumen seems to have "normal" dimensions because the dimensions are the same throughout the vessel length. At autopsy, however, the pathologist sees both the wall and the lumen. There the wall may be shown to be very thickened with diffuse atheromatous disease or with intima or media changes. Although the lumen may have appeared normal to the angiographer, to the pathologist the lumen is narrowed by the percentage of increase of the wall thickness. It is this situation that possibly causes the discrepancy between the angiographic "normal" and the pathologic "abnormal." (Note: This situation shows that we were given good-sized conduits to begin with and can suffer some luminal loss as we age with no symptoms at all.)

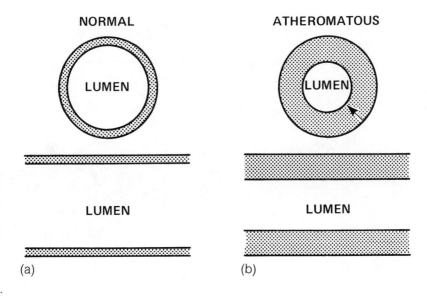

FIGURE 3-8.

Routine Projections and Special Views

BASIC EQUIPMENT

There are numerous types of angiographic rooms for coronary arteriography, varying from simple single-plane to multidirectional C-arms or parallelogram equipment. The most basic need is a single-plane fluororoom with a cut film changer capable of one to two films per second or a room with 16 or 35 mm ciné capability. Although most laboratories now use cineangiograms, one of the main innovators of coronary arteriography, Melvin Judkins, did all his films on serial radiographs. He thought that they were much more accurate than ciné. At present, however, with equipment quality improving by leaps and bounds, almost all laboratories use ciné techniques. With good technical control, superb films can be obtained. Ciné allows multiple frames (30–60 frames per second) and instant viewing on a television tape playback. The last factor allows the angiographer to be certain that he or she has diagnostic film during the procedure.

STANDARD PROJECTIONS

The routine views that should be obtained in all laboratories are a 60-degree LAO and a 35-degree RAO of both coronary arteries. Until a few years ago, most laboratories only expanded this format to include a few more projections around a perpendicular axis, which was the limit of an over-table intensifier with a fixed under-table tube (Figure 4-1). It was these views that we reviewed earlier and will discuss again.

Now, however, new technology has solved one of the major problems once faced in vessel evaluation. The problem involved the three-dimensional aspect of the coronary vessels. Because the vessels cross over and around ventricles, some areas were hidden from the perpendicular beam. For exam-

ple, in the routine LAO in Figure 4-2, the proximal area was impossible to "open up" to an x-ray beam perpendicular to it. Vessel overlap also kept the RAO and lateral views of this area from being diagnostic.

To solve the problem, many laboratories initially repositioned their patients to better visualize the hidden areas. Patients were elevated on a pillow to positions approximately 30 degrees to the fixed perpendicular fluoroscopic equipment (Figures 4-3a and b). The angle allowed a more perpendicular view of vessels that were curved away from the beam when the patient was supine. Figures 4-4a and b give an example of the change in vessel configuration. Note how the lesion at the bifurcation of the septal vessels, and LAD is uncovered.

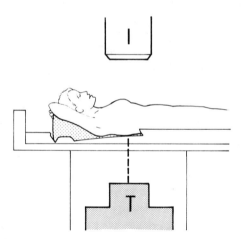

FIGURE 4-1. Patient is supine on the cradle with an under-table tube (T) and overhead intensifier (I). Patient rotates on a cradle under the intensifier. Maximum movement is 45°–60° LAO or RAO.

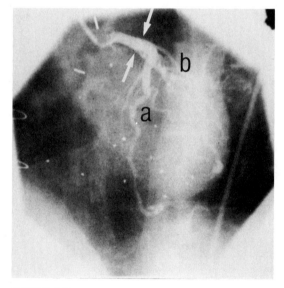

FIGURE 4-2.

CHAPTER 4: ROUTINE PROJECTIONS AND SPECIAL VIEWS

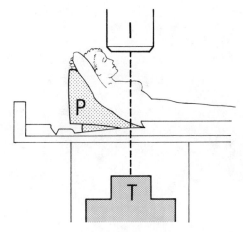

FIGURE 4-3a. The upper trunk of the patient is elevated about 30° onto a preformed radiolucent support (P). This angles the heart so that the beam from tube (T) to intensifier (I) is more perpendicular to the proximal LAD.

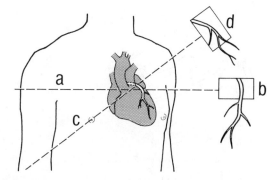

FIGURE 4-3b. A beam (a) perpendicular to the long axis of the body will visualize the proximal portion of the LAD. The vessel is severely foreshortened (b). A beam (c) angled more perpendicular to the area of interest shows the LAD at greater length and improves visualization of the proximal LAD and bifurcating branches (d).

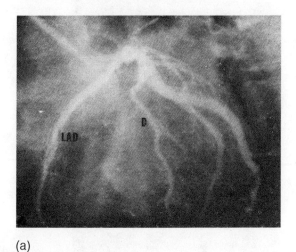

(a)

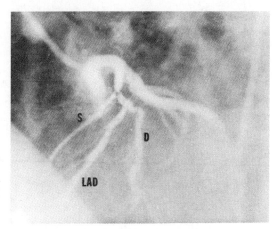

(b)

FIGURE 4-4.

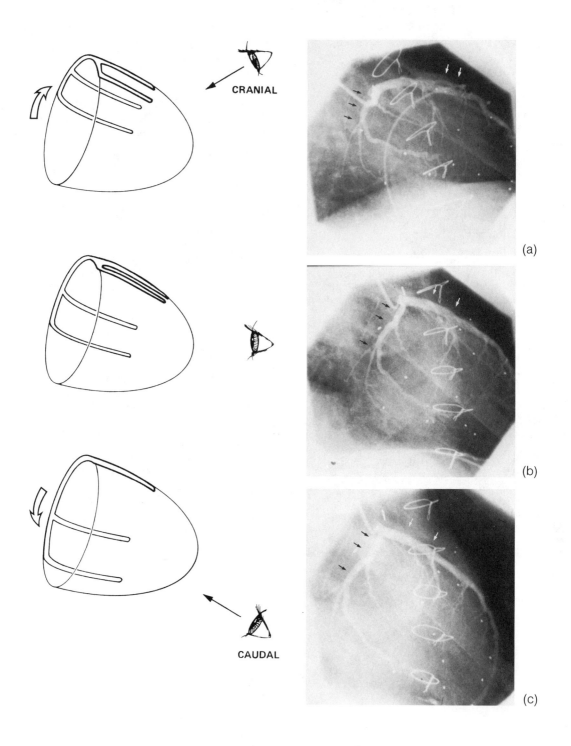

CRANIAL

CAUDAL

(a)

(b)

(c)

In the RAO projection there are different problems, but the angled views are equally beneficial (Figures 4-5a–c). In the RAO projection of the left coronary artery, the problems are at the bifurcation of LAD and circumflex and in the overlap of the diagonals. In the right coronary injection, the problem is with the overlap of the inferior wall vessels. Angling can solve most of these problems.

FIGURE 4-5 (facing page). RAO projections—left coronary. a: Cranial. b: Routine. c: Caudal. In the routine (45°) RAO projection, there are several areas of the vascularity that can be improved through angulation. The small black arrows mark the circumflex system. Comparing the cranial and caudal views to the routine projection, note the shortening of this segment when moving toward the cranial view and the lengthening when moving toward the caudal view. This occurs because of the change in beam direction associated with the rotation. The cranial view rotates the heart clockwise to the beam and the caudal view rotates the heart counterclockwise.

Note in the drawings how the rotation lengthens or shortens the circumflex. The caudal view optimizes the circumflex circulation, particularly in the most proximal portion. The small white arrows mark the LAD and its branches. In the routine projection (b), comparing the drawing to the photo, note how the two anterior vessels depicted on the drawing appear as a single vessel on the photo. These two vessels sit very close to each other and superimpose. On the caudal view they remain superimposed. However, on the cranial view they are separated. The choice of cranial versus caudal for separating these anterior branches depends on how far apart the branches are. If they are well separated, the caudal view often allows excellent visualization with the diagonal vessel appearing below the LAD and above the first marginal. In the present instance, when the diagonal branch is very close to the LAD, the cranial view is successful.

These RAO views need to be used along with the LAO projections. The location of the diagonal branches nearby or well separated from the LAD can be best defined from the LAO views.

C-ARM AND PARALLELOGRAM UNITS

Many catheterization laboratories continue to use this system of placing patients on a pillow. With a variety of LAO and RAO projections, and with the patient on a mobile cradle, these methods are fairly satisfactory. However, most new rooms have been designed to solve the vessel overlap problem with different tube-intensifier configurations. Both parallelogram and C-arm units (Figure 4-6) allow 360-degree rotation around the patient. At the same time, some tube-intensifier units can rotate in cephalad or caudal directions or, if that is not possible, the table can be rotated to the left or right for similar angulations. There are thus numerous additional views that solve the problem of overlap and foreshortening by allowing a more perpendicular orientation to the vessels.

Whatever equipment is available, you will have to acquaint yourself with the routine views and angles used and—most importantly—find out which views maximize which areas. As the ultimate film reader, if you are able to guide the angiographer in filming, you must know what to tell him or her to do.

Figure 4-7 is a chart showing some standard and angulated projections. The drawing assumes use of a C-arm or parallelogram unit with multiple directional movement (rows 2 and 4) or a table move yielding the same projection (rows 3 and 5).

The right side of each block is a diagram from the perspective of someone looking downward at the table. The square is the intensifier; the triangle, the tube. The left diagram is drawn as if seen from the foot of the table. The views are named by the

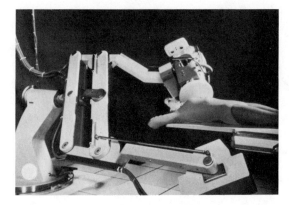

(a)

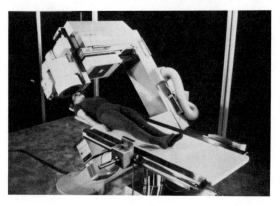

(b)

FIGURE 4-6.

intensifier-heart (*not* the tube-heart) relationship; the top of the heart is cranial, and the bottom of the heart, caudal. Thus, block A-2 is a cranial view because the intensifier relates to the superior aspect of the heart. Although degrees of rotation are given, they are, of course, variable.

Angiographic examples are on the following pages. Review them, comparing them to the routine projections to see the advantages they offer (Figures 4-8–4-12).

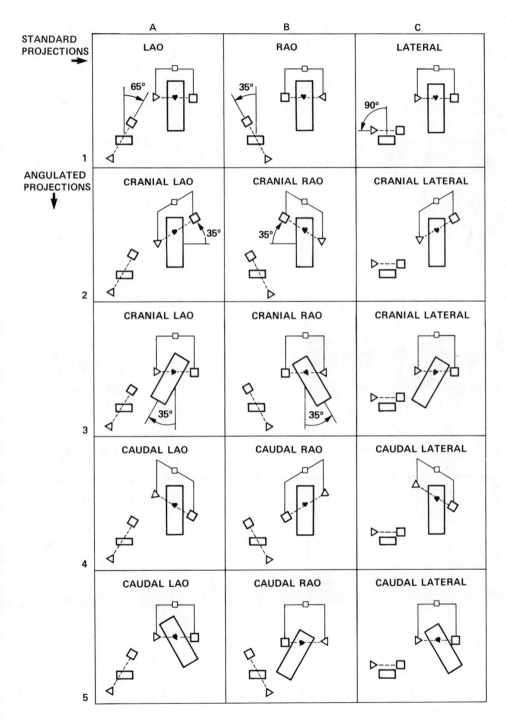

FIGURE 4-7.

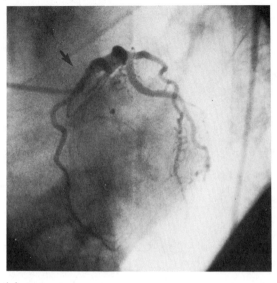

(a)

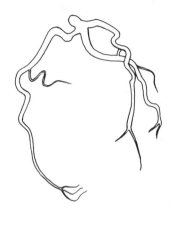

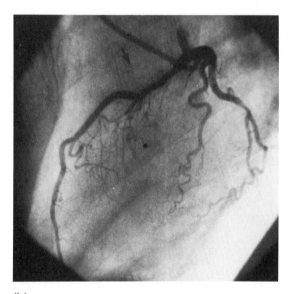

(b)

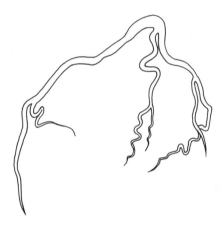

FIGURE 4-8. Left coronary artery injection in LAO projection. a: 60° LAO, no angulation. The arrow indicates the LAD. Note that the vessels are foreshortened proximally and that several of the vessels are bunched together. b: 60° LAO, 30° cranial angulation. Note how cranial angulation elongates the LAD (arrow), moves the high marginal branch away from the proximal circumflex, and allows evaluation of the crucial proximal LAD and circumflex area.

CHAPTER 4: ROUTINE PROJECTIONS AND SPECIAL VIEWS

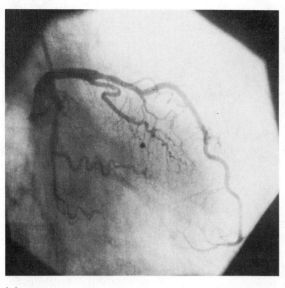
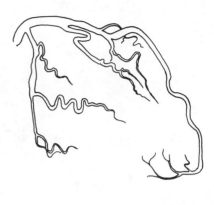

(a)

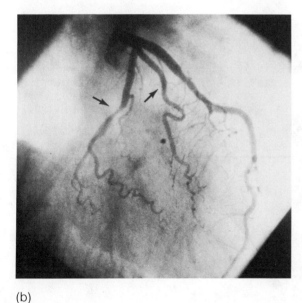
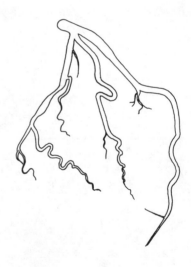

(b)

FIGURE 4-9. Left coronary artery injection in RAO projection. a: 45° RAO, no angulation. Note the foreshortening of the proximal marginal and diagonal branches. b: 45° RAO, 30° caudal angulation. Note how the angulation allows better visualization of these vessels (arrows). A lesion in the circumflex is now well visualized.

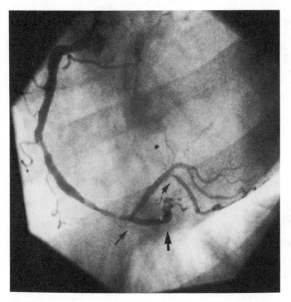

(a)

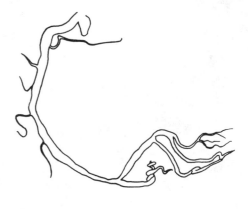

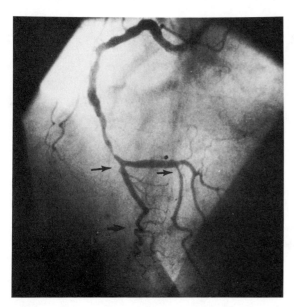

(b)

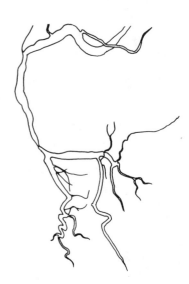

FIGURE 4-10. Right coronary artery injection in LAO projection. a: 45° LAO, no angulation. The arrows illustrate diseased vessels on the inferior wall. The larger arrow points to the foreshortened posterior diagonal artery. b: 45° LAO, 30° cranial angulation. Note how the posterior diagonal artery is lengthened and how the inferior wall bifurcations are better visualized.

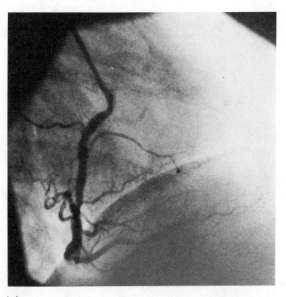

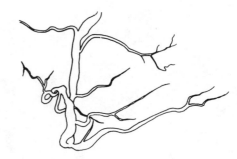

(a)

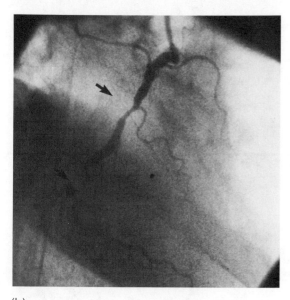

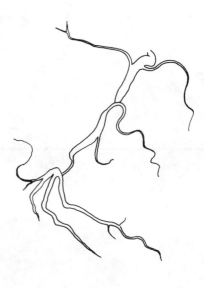

(b)

FIGURE 4-11. Right coronary artery injection in RAO projection. These arteriograms show clearly how improper angulation can mislead the angiographer. a: 45° RAO, no angulation. The main portion of the right coronary artery appears to be well visualized. b: 45° RAO, 30° caudal angulation. Note how the main right coronary artery is opened to view and two severe lesions are revealed (arrows).

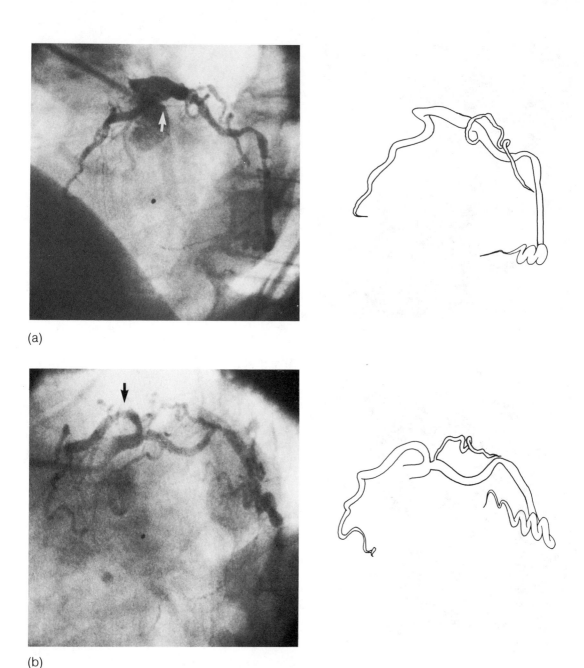

(a)

(b)

FIGURE 4-12. Left coronary artery injection in LAO projection. a: 60° LAO, no angulation. Once again, note the problems with the proximal vessels in this projection (arrows). b: 60° LAO, 30° caudal angulation. This is the "spider view," which moves the proximal LAD and marginal branch superiorly (arrow). This view is particularly useful for viewing the proximal LAD in a transverse heart, in which cranial angulation will not adequately displace the vessel inferiorly.

CHAPTER 5

Collaterals

Collaterals are intervascular connections allowing blood flow from one vessel to another. The stimulus for these connections to form is the need for blood in one area that cannot be supplied in the normal fashion. Whether these connections preexist or form anew is unknown.

The heart develops collateral circulation to generate new blood flow to areas where the flow has been lost or reduced. If collateralization is adequate and develops before myocardium is lost, there may be no symptoms and no muscle death or dysfunction. For good collateralization, there must be both an adequate pathway and adequate time for formation.

But before we go on, one important point must be made: As you progress through this text, it is critical that you know and remember the information of prior sections. To understand collaterals, you must understand normal anatomy. If you do not, go back to Chapter 1 before you go forward.

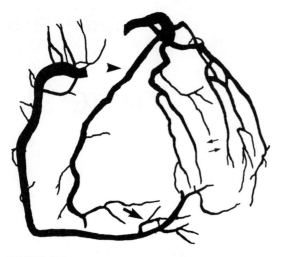

FIGURE 5-1.

COMMON COLLATERALS

Some well-placed vessels in the heart are almost routine collaterals. If these can enlarge, blood flow is often maintained to obstructed vessels. Once again, when there are adequate pathways for collateralization and adequate time for good collaterals to form, symptoms may not occur.

The composite in Figure 5-1 shows the obvious collateral sites. The large arrow shows the potential communication between LAD and PDA, the small arrows between diagonals and marginals, and the arrowhead between right and left proximal arteries.

It will be important for you to note the source and size of collaterals and the vessels that receive distribution from the collaterals. Often, this is the only way that obstructed vessels can be visualized, and decisions for surgery have to be made on the basis of collateral filling.

ADEQUATE PATHWAYS FOR COLLATERALIZATION

Although there are a voluminous number of potential collaterals, you need to remember only a few common ones, which are listed below.

Collaterals fall into two groups: "same side" (left-to-left or right-to-right) and "opposite side" intercoronary collaterals, which may be more important, and in which a branch of the right coronary supplies the left, or vice versa. Same-side collaterals are either one branch to another or "bridging," where small collaterals develop next to a lesion to carry blood distally. The intercoronary types, obviously, are branch-to-branch. There are some classic intercoronary collaterals, and you should note them so that you can search for and identify them.

Some important pathways for collateralization are:

Septal anastomoses. The LAD itself or its septal branches to the PDA or to the LAD from the PDA. Figure 5-2a shows a left injection with collateralization to the PDA through septals from the LAD. Figure 5-2b also shows septal collateral flow, but from the PDA to the obstructed LAD.

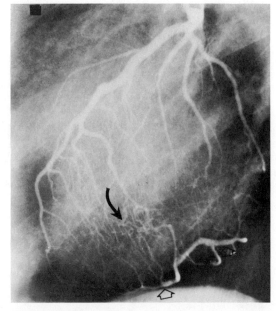

(a)

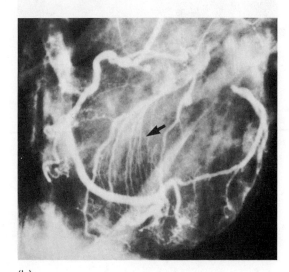

(b)

FIGURE 5-2.

Vieussens ring. Figure 5-3 shows a collateralization from the right coronary artery to the obstructed LAD through the pulmonary conus artery. The curved arrow shows the direction from the right coronary artery through the conus; the LAD is indicated by open arrows.

Inferior wall anastomoses. Distal right to circumflex or circumflex to distal right. Figure 5-4 shows a right injection with collateralization through the distal right coronary artery to left circumflex and marginal branches.

Other, less well known collaterals are:

Kugels anastamoses. Figure 5-5 shows a pathway from the right coronary (closed arrow) through the interventricular branch (open arrows) to AV node to PDA.

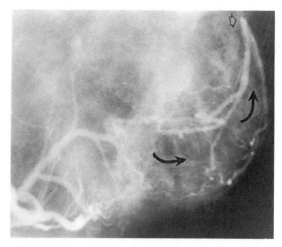

FIGURE 5-4.

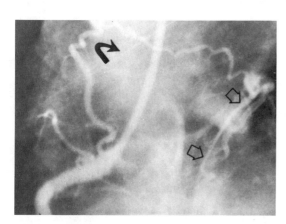

FIGURE 5-3.

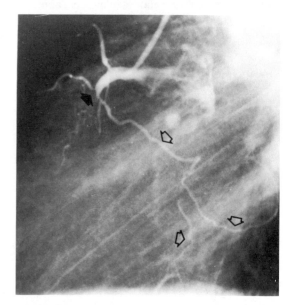

FIGURE 5-5.

Diagonal to marginals. In Figure 5-6, to circumflex. The flow is through epicardial branches (curved arrow).

"Bridging" collaterals. Small branches forming in fatty tissue, usually in the AV groove but occasionally along the LAD. Figure 5-7 shows a proximal-to-mid-right pathway via "bridging" collaterals.

Any other epicardial connection you can imagine, such as the one shown in Figure 5-8, which is a left injection showing collateralization through the atrial branch (closed arrows) to distal right (open arrows).

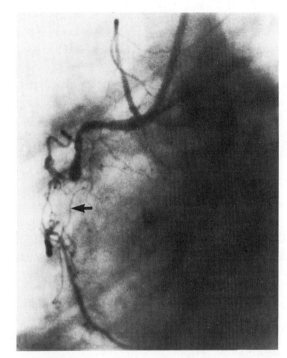

FIGURE 5-7.

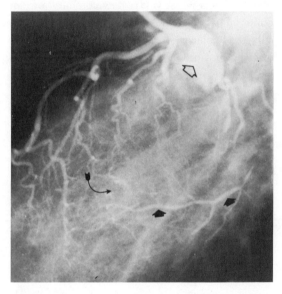

FIGURE 5-6.

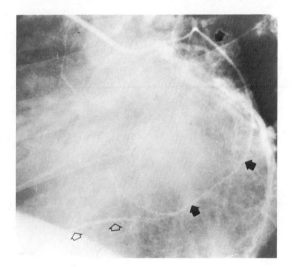

FIGURE 5-8.

These are some of the major collateral pathways. Remember that they are present because of a high-grade significant lesion in the vessel being injected.

An interesting phenomenon occurs when a partially obstructed vessel receives collateral flow—bidirectional flow. Bidirectional flow occurs when pressure distal to a significant lesion is about the same as pressure in the collateral supplying such a vessel. When this occurs, blood is supplied to the distal segment from both native and collateral vessels. When you inject contrast into such a vessel, the flow of contrast to the distal segment is washed away by blood from the collateral vessel. This tells you that though the diseased vessel may have a significant lesion, it is not totally obstructed.

TIME FOR FORMATION

Good collaterals almost announce that the coronary artery lesions have been slowly progressing with gradual loss of blood flow and pressure distal to the lesion. With gradually increasing ischemia as a stimulus, multiple collateral pathways appear to bring needed blood to the area. Pressure in collateral vessels is lower than pressure in normal vessels. Therefore, collateral flow requires a significant lesion in the native vessel—a lesion that creates a fall-off in pressure and flow distal to the obstruction. It is only then that blood can flow from the low pressure collateral system. You will see evidence of this when you review coronary arteriograms on patients who have been operated on with a bypass in place. You will no longer see collaterals once normal pressure is reconstituted in the diseased vessel.

Ventriculography

The purpose of ventriculography is to find out how the ventricle is functioning. The procedure is routinely performed as part of a coronary arterial study or any cardiac study in which left ventricular function is important. In general, the blood entering or already within the heart is opacified with contrast material. Then, with ciné radiographic techniques, multiple images of the heart are obtained as the heart goes through several systolic-diastolic cycles. The ventricle's contractility, its size, the wall thickness, and the quality of valve function are all observed.

VENTRICULAR EVALUATION

Procedure

The heart is usually injected in the 30–45 degree RAO projection, which allows visualization of most of the free wall of the ventricle but not of the ventricular septum and parts of the inferior wall. An LAO ventriculogram, routine or with cranial angulation, along with the RAO projection, will allow evaluation of all walls. If one projection is to be obtained, the RAO is preferred because surgical evaluation is easier in the RAO. The contrast injection into the ventricle usually runs 3–4 seconds and a total of 4–6 systolic-diastolic cycles can usually be evaluated. The number is obviously affected by the heart rate. The study is often performed before coronary arteriography because of the potential effect of the coronary artery injections on myocardial contractility. However, if the patient is very unstable, it is wise to do the coronary arteriograms first and eliminate the ventriculogram if necessary. Functional evaluation of the ventricle can be achieved through nuclear medicine studies or echocardiography.

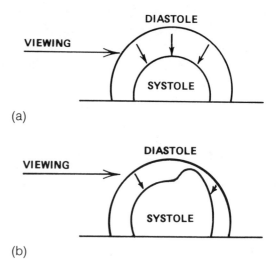

(a)

(b)

FIGURE 6-1.

Contractility

A few notes are necessary as we begin to discuss evaluation of ventriculograms. Figure 6-1 represents a graphic view perpendicular to the free wall of the left ventricle in systole and diastole. This is a representation of the RAO view. Note that this view of the heart does not really show the arcs of the ventricular wall but their summation. Therefore, abnormal segments can be "pulled in" by normal ones, and you would interpret motion as normal. Also, note in Figure 6-1b that normal segments may not be seen in systole because your evaluation is of what "stays out." Thus, the incorrect assumption will be that the whole structure is abnormal.

With these two warnings in mind, let us proceed to how one evaluates the ventricle. Again, a standard nomenclature will make results easy to communicate to others.

We decide on wall motion segment by segment. Note the names of the individual segments in the RAO projection (Figure 6-2a): two basal—anterior and posterior (numbers 1 and 5); apical (number 3); diaphragmatic (number 4); and anterolateral (number 2).

Even though the LAO view will be used less often, it is important to realize that the two views are complementary, not exclusive. Though less often used, the evaluation will be the same, but the segments are of course different. In Figure 6-2b, numbers 6 and 7 evaluate the septum, and 8, 9, and 10, the "other side" of the RAO, the posterior, inferior, and superior lateral segments. The primary evaluation in observing ventricular function is for motion, since function is correlated with how well the walls move. Remember, be careful not to be too sophisti-

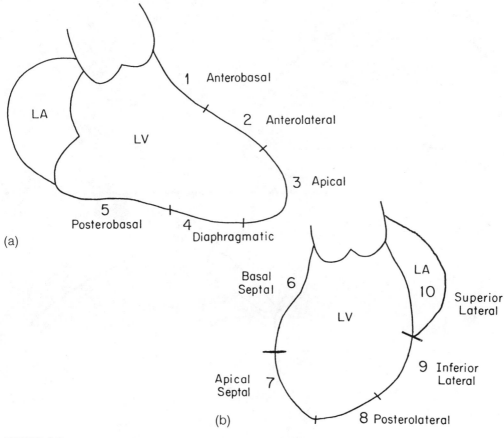

FIGURE 6-2.

cated with your language. Your choices of nomenclature for each segment are:

Normal (Figure 6-3). If the ventricle has normal contractility, all segments move normally. All segments move toward a central point fairly equally, although any one segment may move more than a perceived norm. The norm is usually eyeballed, but if the motion was measured (planimetered), the area difference in the ventricle between systole and diastole would show that 50% or more of the diastolic volume had disappeared during systole. This, of course, represents the normal ejection volume of the ventricle. (Note that the same volume

could be ejected with abnormal wall motion. One area moves abnormally and a second area moves excessively to compensate for it. Therefore, the ejection volume could remain the same.) "Normal" means normal wall motion segmentally, but a normal ventricle obviously has a 50% or greater area change as well.

Hypokinesia (Figure 6-4). Note the decreased inward motion in the anterobasal, diaphragmatic, and apical segments. You can, if you trace systole and diastole atop each other on a piece of paper as we have in Figures 6-3 and 6-4, discern whether the movement is mildly or severely decreased. The effort will also give you some practical experience on which to build your visual accuracy. You can thus evaluate this motion subjectively or, if you wish to trace the chambers, objectively.

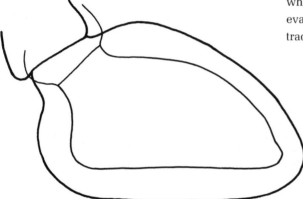

FIGURE 6-3.

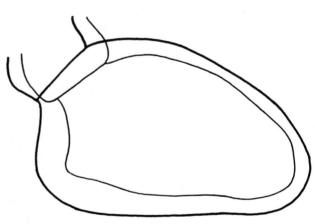

FIGURE 6-4.

CHAPTER 6: VENTRICULOGRAPHY

Akinesia (Figure 6-5). No motion is shown in the anterolateral segment. Anterobasal and apical hypokinesia is apparent.

Dyskinesia (Figure 6-6). Unusual wall motion of any kind. The motion can be inward but may be unusual because of timing. This is sometimes seen when there is a conduction abnormality but more often is unexplained. In Figure 6-6, the unusual motion is outward in systole rather than inward. This type of dyskinesia is called *paradoxical motion* and is usually due to *aneurysm* formation.

Ventricular aneurysms are thin-walled sections of nonvital myocardium.

Because of various tube-intensifier distances, magnification modes, and nonstandardized degrees of rotation that are used in different laboratories, most laboratories develop their own values for chamber size and ejection volume by standardizing their factors and developing a regression formula to handle variations in rotation, size, magnification, and so on. These findings can be put into a computer; through the use of a light pen, the ventriculogram can be outlined on the TV screen and rapid calculation of volumes achieved. A fairly accurate quantitative measurement can be achieved with this technique.

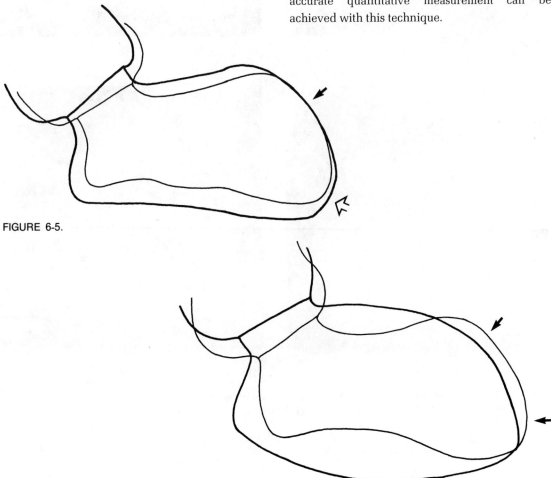

FIGURE 6-5.

FIGURE 6-6.

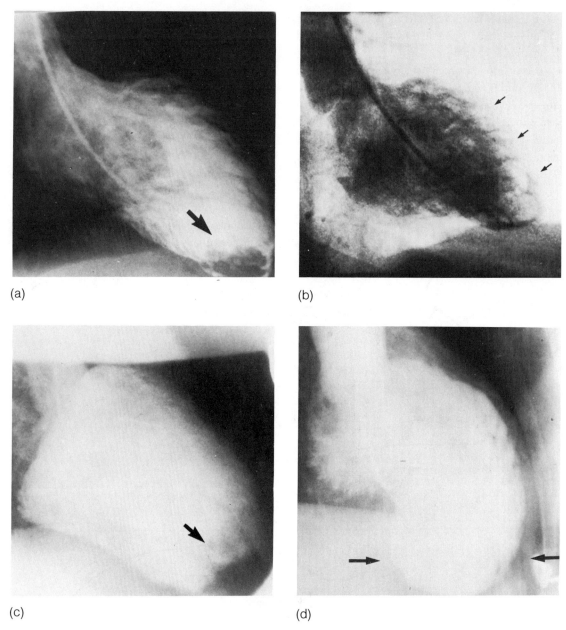

FIGURE 6-7. a: Thrombus at apex. b: Multiple thrombi, anterolateral. c: Irregular thrombus with "squaring off" of apex. d: Large aneurysmal dilatation.

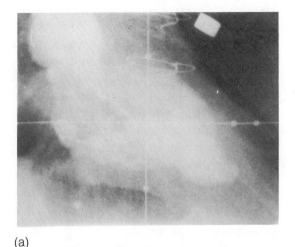

(a)

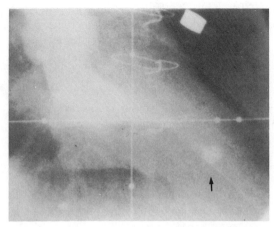

(b)

A more common alternative is to eyeball the chamber. Since you will be familiar with your own laboratory equipment, your judgment will probably be correct. But if you are evaluating a study from another laboratory, be wary.

Chamber configuration and content should also be mentioned if it is unusual. The chamber may be unusually smooth-walled or excessively trabeculated. It may be globular and thin-walled or hypertrophic and thick-walled. There may be single or multiple filling defects—smooth or irregular, round or sharp-edged. Figures 6-7 and 6-8 show examples of some of these irregularities.

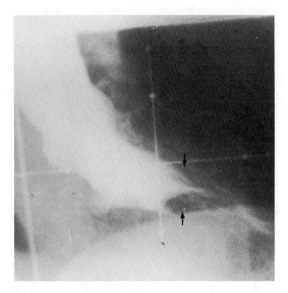

(c)

FIGURE 6-8a–c. Diastole to systole in hypercontractile ventricle. The arrow in b indicates contrast in small apical area separated from remainder of ventricular due to hypercontractility. Arrows in c point to large papillary muscles.

WALL THICKNESS

Wall thickness should be evaluated during diastole (Figure 6-9). It can be done when a surface vessel, the myocardial wall, and the ventricular chamber appear simultaneously on the same plane. Again, there are no absolute measurements for wall thickness because of the variation in projection, magnification, and radiographic equipment. You will learn the normal variation with experience.

In the RAO projection, wall thickness can be evaluated in a view of the inferior wall when the posterior descending artery, the myocardium, and the inferior ventricular chamber appear at once. The anterior wall is impossible to use because the vessels are not necessarily in proper spatial relationship to the portion of the chamber you are visualizing. Also, the right ventricle may be on the same visual plane as the left ventricle.

VALVE FUNCTION

A check of valve calcification, valve motion, and competency is the final part of ventricular evaluation. Although valve function is based on hemodynamic measurement, a portion of the mitral and aortic valves appear in the RAO projections and should be commented upon. Several aspects can be evaluated: calcification, valve motion, and valve competency.

Calcification

Either valve may be calcified, as well as the valve rings or the aortic root wall. The quantity of calcium on the valve leaflets often relates directly to the severity of the disease process involved. Fluoroscopy usually shows calcification well, and the motion or configuration defines the location of the calcification. For our purposes, it will suffice to say that valve calcification will have significant motion if the calcification is on mobile valve leaflets. Though aortic and mitral valve calcification can be confused in the RAO projection, rotating to the LAO will separate the valves and allow proper identification.

Valve Motion

In the RAO projection, the posterior leaf of the mitral valve appears tangentially and can be followed throughout its cycle. Figure 6-10 shows an example of such movement. If the posterior leaf opens normally, one can assume that there is no mitral stenosis. It is not necessary to see both leaflets to reach this conclusion. A similar assumption holds true for the aortic valve. In the RAO projection, the left and

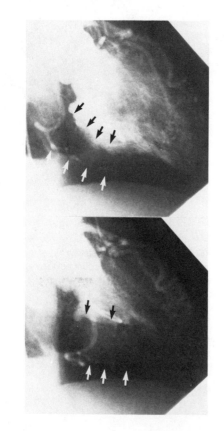

(a)

(b)

FIGURE 6-9. a: Diastole. b: Systole. Black arrows mark the inferior wall of the ventricular cavity. White arrows mark the posterior descending artery (PDA). The space between the two markers is the left ventricular wall. Note the increased thickness in systole compared to diastole. The evaluation should be made in *diastole*.

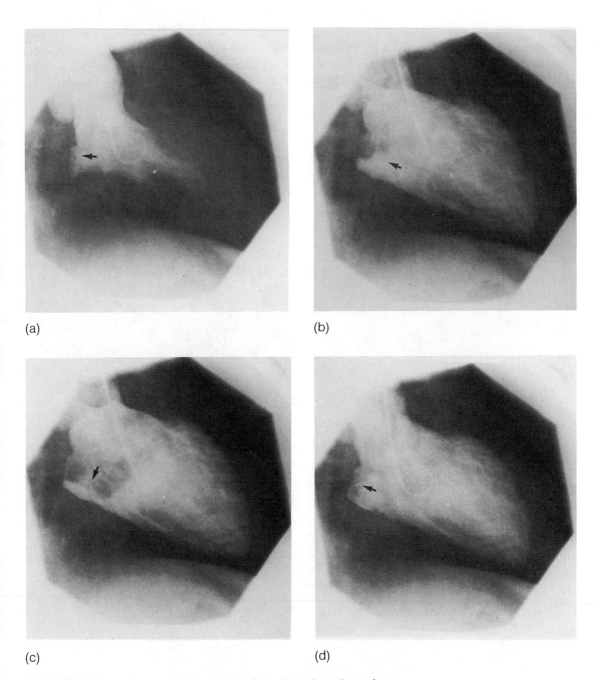

FIGURE 6-10. This series reveals isolated motion of the mitral valve as it goes from the fully closed position in a, the intermediate position in b, the full opened position in c, and back to the closed position in d. Note that the valve is seen because of radiolucent blood flowing against a collection of contrast trapped behind the valve during ventricular diastole.

right cusps are not seen. Only the noncoronary cusp appears tangentially (Figure 6-11). Because disease retarding normal valve motion starts at the wall and works centrally along all of the commissures, if one leaflet is abnormal, usually all leaflets are abnormal (in that they do not open entirely). If the valves open abnormally, they are seen to "dome" [Figures 6-12a (aortic) and b (mitral)].

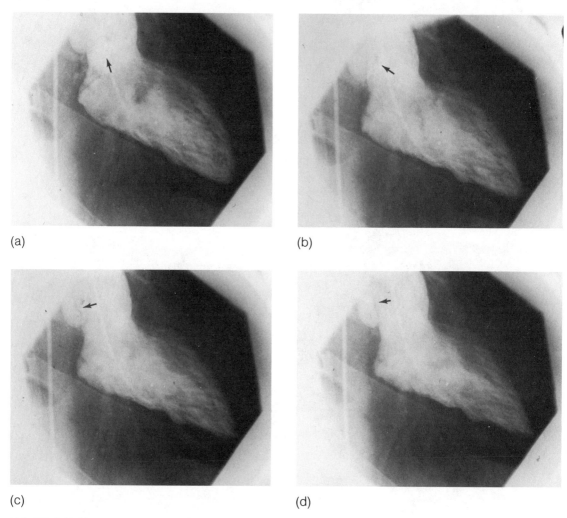

(a)

(b)

(c)

(d)

FIGURE 6-11. This series show the motion of the aortic valve as it goes from its fully closed position in a to its fully open position in d. Note that the valve leaflet is thin and straight in its final open position.

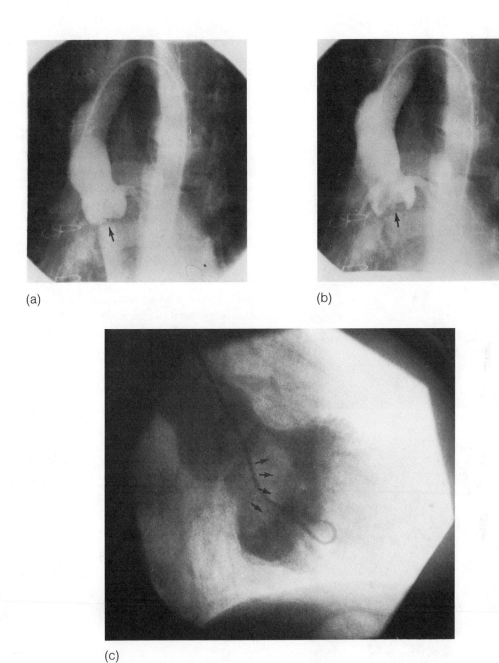

(a)

(b)

(c)

FIGURE 6-12. a, b: The aortic valve in its closed position and in its open domed position in a patient with aortic stenosis. Note how the valve curves centrally, essentially narrowing down the effective orifice. In c, particularly using the prior normal mitral valve opening for comparison, you can see the mitral valve dome as radiolucent blood rushes into the ventricle from the atrium.

Valve Competency

In evaluating valve competency, we are trying to determine the amount of blood regurgitating from the left ventricle to the left atrium on a left ventricular injection or from the aorta to the left ventricle on aortic injection. The volume of regurgitation should be judged similarly for both aortic and mi-

tral valves. After the injection is over, the observer can evaluate the amount of regurgitation according to the following criteria (1+–4+):

- Trace or slight amount of contrast in left atrium or left ventricle
- Atrium or ventricle filled but not staying filled for three beats
- Less dense than the proximal chamber but lasting longer than three beats
- Denser or equal density with the ventricle or aorta and lasting greater than three beats

When evaluating for regurgitation, be sure to observe the valve leaflets, which may define abnormal motion or thickness as a potential cause. Try also to observe whether the regurgitant jet is central or peripheral, again attempting to define a cause (paravalvular leaks, asymmetric jets due to valve prolapse with papillary muscle rupture, and so on) (Figure 6-13).

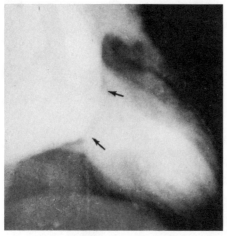

(a)

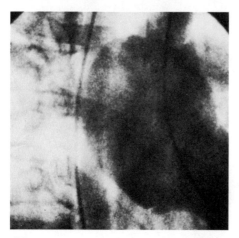

(b)

FIGURE 6-13. Both and and b frames evidence high grade (4+) mitral regurgitation. In a, the arrows point to a thickened mitral valve in a patient with mitral stenosis and mitral regurgitation. Note the discordance between the atrial size and the ventricular size. This usually means that mitral stenosis is longer-standing than the mitral regurgitation.

THE VENTRICULOGRAM REPORT

To summarize, after evaluating the ventricle, you should be able to comment on size, contractility, chamber description, and valve motion and competency. Table 6-1 shows the information you would give in a ventriculogram report.

TABLE 6-1   A Ventriculogram Report

Function
Size
Contractility
Wall thickness
Valve function
Ejection volume
Normal/enlarged
Normal/hypokinetic/akinetic/dyskinetic
Normal/thin/thick
Normal/stenosed/regurgitant

Vessel Motion

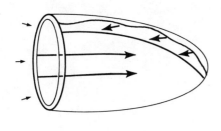

(a)

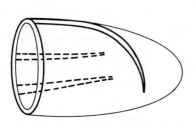

(b)   **DIASTOLE**

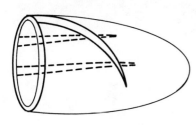

(c)   **SYSTOLE**

FIGURE 7-1.

Now that you have covered vessel anatomy and ventricular function, I have a bonus section for you that, with your new knowledge, will help with vessel location and evaluation.

First, you must accept the notion not only that the ventricle contracts apex toward base, but that there is a rotary motion of the lateral wall. Pick up the model and once again review the positions of the major vessels. You should first hold the model LAO to identify the LAD, diagonal, marginal, and circumflex arteries. Then, rotate the model to RAO to see the new location of each vessel. Figure 7-1 depicts the mitral ring (small arrows) and particularly the lateral free wall of the ventricle (long arrows) moving to the right (toward the apex) during ventricular systole. The medium arrows represent the interventricular groove and the LAD, which move to the base during systole. Thus, Figure 7-1b (diastole) and Figure 7-1c (systole) show how the LAD seems to cross the lateral wall vessels during ventricular systole.

With that in mind, consider Figures 7-2 through 7-9. This series is aimed at defining the location and motion of four important vessels in LAO and RAO projections. If you understand these four, movement of all the other vessels will make sense. The ciné frames in Figures 7-2 and 7-3 show the left coronary injection in the LAO and RAO projections in diastole (a) and systole (b). The vessels are lettered as LAD (A), diagonal (B), marginal (C), and circumflex (D).

These ciné frames illustrate the motion of each of these vessels in each view.

Figure 7-4 shows a tracing of the four vessels in the LAO and RAO positions in diastole. The composite, Figure 7-5 (page 66), summarizes the movement of vessels from diastole to systole. Location during diastole is indicated by a solid line, location during systole by a dotted line.

Facing page: FIGURE 7-2a, b, top; FIGURE 7-3a, b, middle; FIGURE 7-4a, b, bottom.

CHAPTER 7: VESSEL MOTION

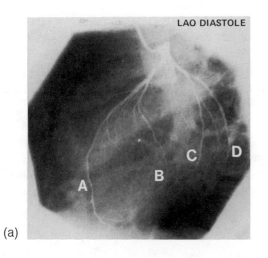

LAO DIASTOLE

(a)

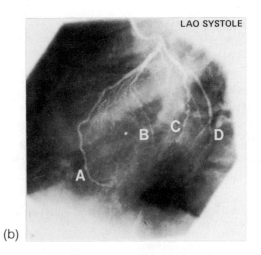

LAO SYSTOLE

(b)

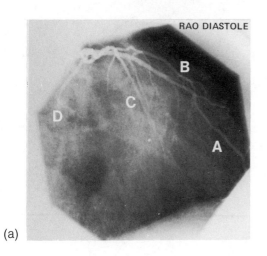

RAO DIASTOLE

(a)

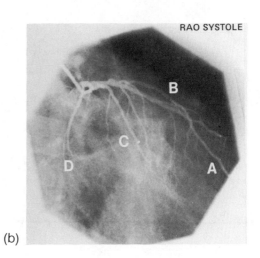

RAO SYSTOLE

(b)

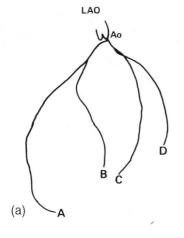

LAO

(a)

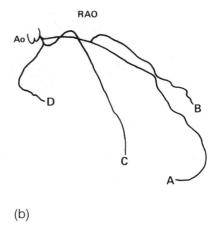

RAO

(b)

Figure 7-6 shows the LAO and RAO views of the LAD and motion in systole. Note that in both views the LAD moves from apex to base.

Figure 7-7 shows that in the LAO, the diagonal branch moves similarly to the LAD, but in the RAO it moves opposite to the LAD. Figure 7-8 shows that in the LAO, the marginal branch moves toward the LAD, but in the RAO view it also moves opposite to the LAD. Note that in the RAO view, the diagonals and marginals move opposite to the LAD because of the rotary motion of the lateral wall, where they reside. It is for this reason that the LAD and lateral wall vessels seem to cross during systole. They are obviously on different walls, moving in opposite directions, to appear this way. (The other vessels that will appear to cross are septal branches, on the same linear plane as the LAD, routinely appearing crossed by lateral wall vessels.)

Figure 7-9 shows that in the LAO, the circumflex branch moves toward the LAD in systole. The apex and base approach each other during systolic contraction. In the RAO, since the circumflex branch resides in the AV groove at the base of the heart, it moves toward the apex.

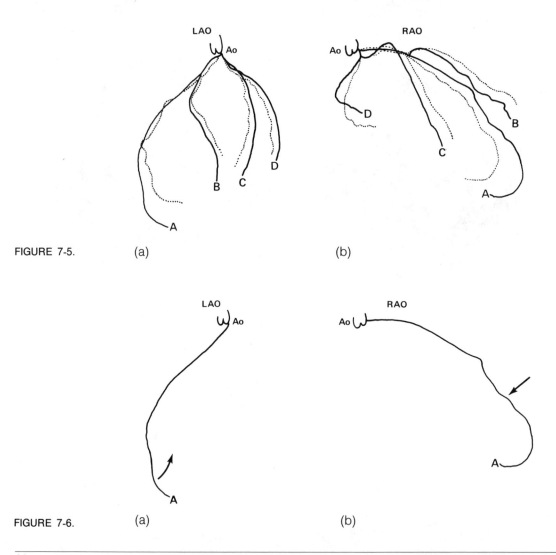

FIGURE 7-5.   (a)   (b)

FIGURE 7-6.   (a)   (b)

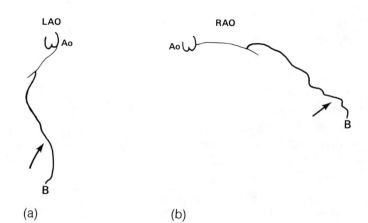

FIGURE 7-7. (a) (b)

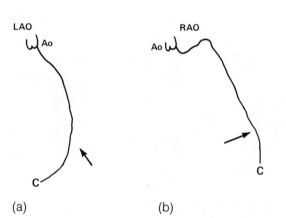

FIGURE 7-8. (a) (b)

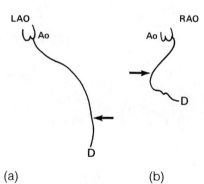

FIGURE 7-9. (a) (b)

After reviewing the movement of these vessels in these two views, you should not confuse the LAD for either marginal or diagonal, even though these two vessels may be very close to the LAD location in the RAO view. From this exercise, you can see how an LAD absent in the LAO projection (cover vessel A with your hand or a piece of paper) could seem to be present in the RAO. The vessel appearing in the RAO in the area of the LAD would be a marginal or a diagonal. But the movement of these vessels in systole should tip you off, as should the absence of a vessel in the LAD area on the LAO.

Coronary Artery Bypass Grafts

Clinical studies have shown that about 80%–85% of the patients who undergo coronary artery bypass grafting have relief of symptoms. Long-term studies of patients with bypass grafts reveal a high percentage of grafts remaining patent for more than five years after the procedure with the yearly closure rate approximately 10%. Although the results have been excellent and the number of patients undergoing the surgery has burgeoned, a reasonable number of patients experience early or late return of symptoms. Grafts can close or narrow—early often because of surgical problems or late because of fibrosis or atherosclerotic change within the venous graft. If symptoms return, patients are sent back to the catheterization lab for reevaluation. Part of that evaluation is to inject the grafts.

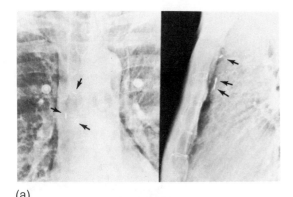

(a)

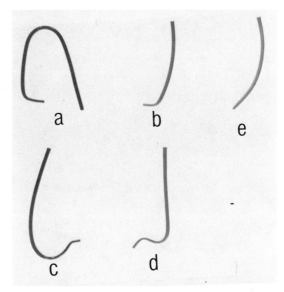

(b)

FIGURE 8-1. a: PA and lateral radiographs in a post-graft patient. The clips are marked with small black arrows and are at the aortic origins of the grafts. In the PA view, the right sided clip marks the right coronary graft, the most superior clip the circumflex, and the lower mid clip, the LAD graft. On the lateral view, the location of the origins on the anterior aorta is clearly indicated by the clip positions. b: An interoperative photo showing a right graft (open arrow), LAD graft (closed arrow), and circ-marginal graft (curved arrow).

In many, but not all, hospitals the surgeons mark the graft origin sites with small rings or clips (Figure 8-1a). Because the grafts tend to be placed in the same locations, the markers, though useful, are not strictly necessary. The right coronary grafts usually emanate along the right midlateral aorta, above the right coronary sinus. The left grafts are anterior on the aorta, with the LAD graft usually the lowest. Note in Figure 8-1b, an intraoperative photo, the common location of such origins. It should be noted that special catheters are often needed for these studies (Figure 8-2). Amplatz right coronary catheters of varying sizes are very useful for left grafts. A

FIGURE 8-2. a: Judkins left catheter. b: Judkins right catheter. c: Amplatz left catheter. d: Amplatz right catheter. e: Wexler catheter.

Wexler graft catheter is often used for right grafts. This catheter is similar to a Judkins right catheter, but the tip is turned downward to better enter the graft. The Amplatz catheter is also excellent for searching the anterior wall of the aorta (Figure 8-3.)

A graft study must show the aortic origin, the full length of the graft, and the anastomosis to the native vessel. The remainder of the native vessel must be studied to eliminate additional lesions. Figures 8-4 to 8-7 are examples of graft injections.

If a graft cannot be found, often the stump is entered with the catheter. (Documentation is important.) If the vessel is not located, an aortogram should be done to rule out the presence of a patent graft. If the right graft is not found, an aortogram should be performed in an LAO projection. If the left-sided grafts are not located, an aortogram must be done in the RAO projection (Figure 8-8).

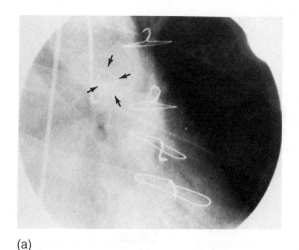 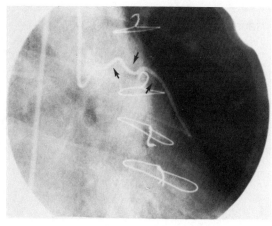

(a)   (b)

FIGURE 8-3. RAO projections of graft injections. a: RAO injections of aorto-coronary graft. A metallic ring (black arrows) has been placed around the graft origin at surgery. An Amplatz graft catheter is in position. b: Injection of contrast into the graft. Small arrows mark the vein in its proximal portion.

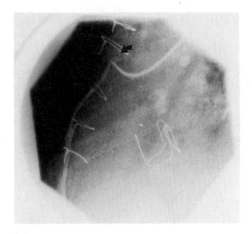

(a)

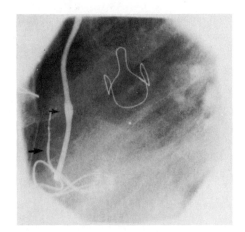

(b)

FIGURE 8-4. a: Injection of the right coronary graft in the LAO projection. Note the reflux of contrast out of the graft ostia. The patient had a heterograft aortic valve replacement. One can use the location of the aortic valve stent to find the right coronary ostia. You can also find the usual location of the origin of the right graft above the right coronary sinus of the valsalva. b: The right coronary graft in the lateral projection. Note the swelling in the graft, which represents a valve (small arrow). Note also the retrograde filling of the native vessel (large arrow). c: An injection of the native right coronary in the RAO projection. The small arrow points to the bypassed lesion. Note the retrograde filling of the graft (large arrow).

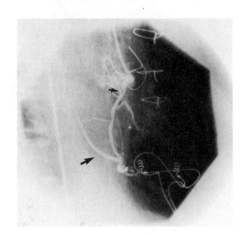

(c)

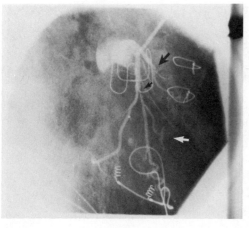
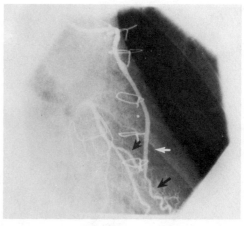

(a)   (b)

FIGURE 8-5. a: Injection of native left coronary artery. Note the bypassed
marginal artery lesion (small arrow) and flash filling of small portion of graft (white
arrow). Note also that the stump of the LAD is seen. b: Injection of graft shows
antegrade and retrograde filling of the left system. This projection is a steeper
RAO, but the bypassed marginal lesion can still be seen.

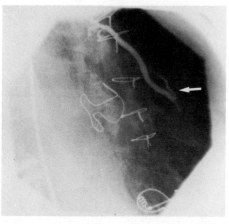
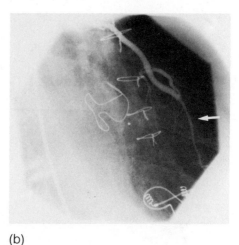

(a)   (b)

FIGURE 8-6. a: Injection of graft to LAD: ostia, full length, and insertion of graft
(small arrow). b: Remainder of vessel is seen later in the injection. As flow down
grafts is often slow, the filming time may need to be prolonged.

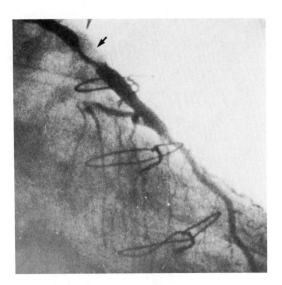

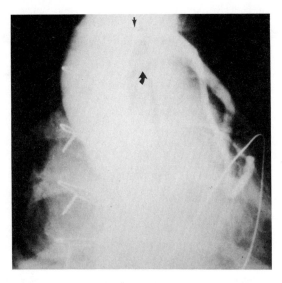

FIGURE 8-7. Graft to LAD. Note the long, narrowed segment (arrow). This is a common type of lesion seen in grafts, often close to the origin from the aorta or insertion into the native vessel. Pathology usually shows intimal overgrowth.

FIGURE 8-8. Aortogram in the AP projection reveals grafts to LAD and circumflex. If the graft origins cannot be found, an aortogram is indicated. Once the grafts are seen and localized, further attempts to catheterize the grafts will probably be successful.

CHAPTER 8: CORONARY ARTERY BYPASS GRAFTS

CHAPTER 9

Technical Considerations

Many of you may never actually perform a coronary arteriogram or a ventriculogram. However, for those who may, or for those who are interested, this chapter is a short summary of technical factors. Personally, I feel that even though a physician may only interpret a study, an understanding of methods and techniques is most important.

CATHETERS

Several catheter systems are available for coronary arteriography. Catheterization is most often done through the femoral artery, but the brachial approach is occasionally used if there is an obstruction in the iliofemoral system or if the presence of excessive aortic tortuosity would lead to loss of catheter control. An alternative to the brachial approach is a percutaneous axillary approach, which allows the use of femoral catheter systems.

One of the original systems, the Sones method, uses a multihole catheter that is inserted through a brachial artery cutdown. The same catheter is manipulated into both coronary arteries and the ventricle. The technique requires a good deal of training and skill, but even with good skills, a certain number of studies end with a lost brachial pulse.

A currently popular method is the Judkins technique (Figure 9-1 a,b). This technique uses a percutaneous femoral puncture and necessitates inserting first a left (Figure 9-1a) and then a right (Figure 9-1b) preformed coronary catheter. These catheters can be either 7 or 8 French and are curved in relation to the width of the aortic root. Manipulation of these catheters is fairly simple and can be learned rather quickly. Each of these catheters has only an end hole through which contrast is injected, and between injections, the end hole is the sole source of pressure measurement. As this is the only hole, as long as normal pressure is measurable, the operator is assured the catheter is not obstructing the vessel.

Because multiple holes are necessary to deliver contrast at speeds required for good chamber visualization, ventriculography requires the insertion of a pigtail catheter into the ventricle (Figure 9-2). The pigtail catheter can be inserted and ventriculography performed before or after coronary arteriograms are obtained.

Although many catheters are available, the only other method I would like to mention is the Amplatz catheter system. Like the Judkins technique, the Amplatz catheter is inserted percutaneously by femoral artery puncture, and the catheters are also sized relative to the aortic root anatomy. Often, just one catheter can be used for both left and right coronary arteries. Again, a separate pigtail catheter must be inserted to perform the ventriculogram. Right Amplatz catheters are excellent for studying grafts. The left Amplatz catheter (9-1c) is often used when the aortic root is very wide.

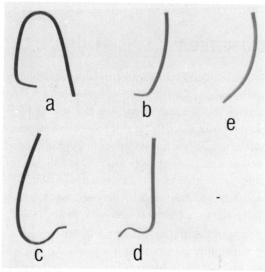

FIGURE 9-1.

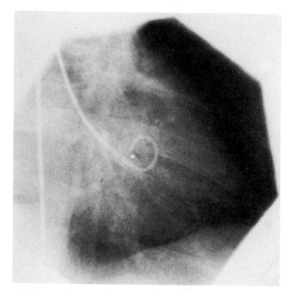

FIGURE 9-2.

CONTRAST MATERIAL

The contrast material we generally use is 66% diatrizoate meglumine and 10% diatrizoate sodium. The iodine concentration must be adequate for good visualization. When studying the heart, it is important to use a contrast material that has a long history of safety. Otherwise, significant arrhythmias may occur related to the electrolyte mixture in the solution.

INJECTION

Electrocardiographic and Pressure Changes

Following injection of the coronary arteries there are routine electrocardiographic findings, with T-wave changes the most dramatic (Figure 9-3a). Slowing of the heart rate is also common. Since these findings should return to normal between injections, you should wait for return to baseline before continuing the injection series. The reversion toward normal usually occurs momentarily and moves quickly toward the preinjection tracing. Systolic pressure also falls and quickly returns to normal between injections (Figure 9-3b). This finding is also routine and should not cause alarm unless pressure remains low. If it does, immediate removal of the catheter from the coronary orifice is mandatory. Usually, the catheter has advanced and the end hole has moved against the vessel wall, damping the pressure. However, occasionally the catheter obstructs the vessel lumen and this potential occurrence is what really demands rapid catheter removal. We have patients give a short cough after each injection. The cough is effective in raising pressure and increasing the heart rate when there are slightly long periods of bradycardia.

Injection Volume and Speed

Nowhere is injection speed more critical to good visualization and safety than in the coronary artery. Because of coronary arterial pulsatile blood flow, with the greatest forward flow during diastole and the backward flow with reflux during ventricular systole, a major effort needs to be made to get a good contrast bolus with each injection. This is easier with 8 French than 7 French catheters and is particularly difficult in large volume hearts or during studies of hearts with rapid rhythms. A few laboratories use a mechanical injector system to guarantee appropriate speed and volume. In our laboratory we do all injections by hand. We prefer to use plastic syringes rather than glass because the sticky contrast material does not make them jam; I feel that they allow a faster injection rate. Contrast volume is approximately 6–8 mL per injection. Though it lessens contrast for vessel visualization, reflux from the coronary artery back into the aorta is mandatory to evaluate for ostial lesions.

VENTRICULOGRAPHY

A pigtail catheter is usually used in ventriculography, as was mentioned previously. The catheter should be placed with the pigtail near the base of the ventricle, not touching the ventricular wall. The position will prevent extra systoles during injection and is worth taking time to achieve, for a sustained arrhythmia often occurs during the injection and negates the value of the study. Occasional irregular beats can be controlled with a 50–75 mg bolus of lidocaine just before injection of contrast. The volume of contrast for the ventriculogram should be 40–50 mL injected at 10–12 mL/sec. This will give good opacification and will rarely cause irritability. Some laboratories inject at a faster rate and achieve better opacification; however, this practice is more likely to cause extra systoles during the ventriculogram. Four side holes are adequate to opacify the ventricle. The addition of more side holes only means more vigorous flushing to keep the most proximal ones (furthest from the end hole) clear of thrombus.

The value of anticoagulation before coronary arteriography has been accepted by many laboratories. The method is to administer heparin after placement of the arterial catheter. (We use 45–50 units/kg.) After completing the study, we inject a similar quantity of protamine to reverse the heparin effect. Heparin in also used in the flushing solution during the procedure.

Some think that this anticoagulation procedure has prevented many of the embolic phenomena and thrombosis that have occurred at the catheter insertion site. In some laboratories the number of hematomas following the procedure has increased slightly. Coagulation studies should be obtained beforehand, if indicated, as with all angiographic procedures. Although the urgency of the procedure must be the driving factor, hematologic advice should be obtained if there is any blood factor abnormality.

PACING

Some laboratories routinely insert a pacemaker before every study. We often insert pacers when resting heart rates are less than 60 or if the patient has left bundle branch block (LBBB); right bundle branch block (RBBB) sometimes occurs during the study and inserting a pacer in a patient with LBBB protects against the hazard of complete heart block.

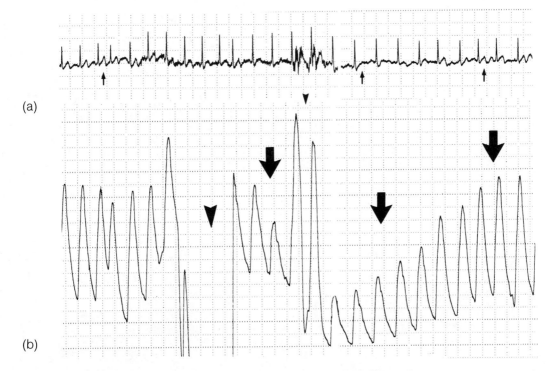

(a)

(b)

FIGURE 9-3. Electrocardiograph and pressure tracing during coronary arteriography. a: ECG strip recorded during injection. Small black arrows (left) marks normal T waves prior to injection, (middle) T waves flattening immediately after injection, and (right) return of T waves 3–5 beats later. b: Pressure tracing simultaneous with ECG. Drop in pressure marked by large arrowhead indicates the injection. Since pressure is measured via the catheter end hole, there is no pressure measurement during the injection. The first pressure wave after injection is the same as the pre-injection level. The large black arrows indicate falling pressure after injection with gradual rise back to normal baseline. The two high-pressure spikes marked by the small arrowhead occur during the post-injection cough, which the patient is asked to perform after each injection.

CHAPTER 10

Drugs Used in Coronary Arteriography

Numerous drugs are used during coronary arteriography, but I will mention only a few of the more common ones:

Atropine. Atropine is often used during angiography if there are arrhythmias that respond to it. It should be noted that many laboratories use atropine prophylactically before study to reduce vagal attacks. We do not and have encountered no problems treating a reaction when it does occur. The issue is whether to treat many patients for a problem that occurs in few.

Nitroglycerin. Nitroglycerin is also used routinely during angiography whenever an anginal episode occurs. A sublingual dose usually quickly rids the patient of the angina. However, parenteral nitroglycerin can be used when necessary, intravenously or, on occasion, by intracoronary injection.

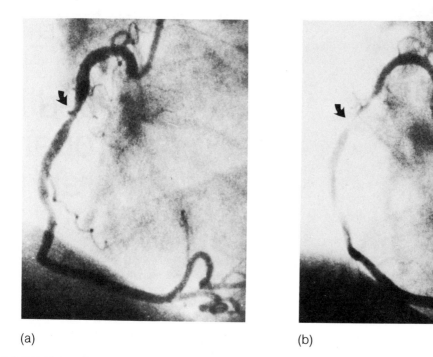

(a)   (b)

FIGURE 10-1. a: Right coronary injection in LAO projection. Arrows mark lesion. b: Following ergonovine injection. Note how high grade the proximal artery has become. This change was accompanied by pain and ECG change.

Heparin-Protamine. We routinely anticoagulate our patients. Once the arterial line is in, we administer 50 units of heparin per kilogram of body weight. Our flushing solutions also contain heparin (2 units of heparin per milliliter of flush solution). The initial heparin bolus plus routine flushing keeps the anticoagulation level adequate. At the termination of the procedure, we reverse the anticoagulation with protamine. There have been no major problems with this procedure, although there may be a slight increase in the incidence of small hematomas.

Ergonovine Maleate. This drug, as well as a few others, is very effective in eliciting coronary artery spasm in patients being tested for susceptibility. The positive reactors are usually patients with atypical (Prinzmetal) angina, and sometimes the response can be truly remarkable, with normal vessels markedly narrowed or no longer visualized (Figure 10-1). These findings are usually rapidly reversed with nitroglycerin, but, because occasional patients are unresponsive, ergonovine should be used with caution. The drug has been used most often in patients with atypical angina but is now increasingly used in patients whose clinical symptoms seem to be disproportionate to their degree of coronary artery disease. The yield in patients with non-Prinzmetal angina is rather small. Patients must be selected carefully for this regimen.

Streptokinase. Streptokinase is a potent thrombolytic agent that is administered intravenously or by intracoronary injection to dissolve fresh thrombi. If it is used within the early hours of thrombosis, myocardial salvage is often possible as the blockage dissolves. Some consider the procedure to be of value because bypass grafting or balloon dilatation of underlying disease is possible following the streptokinase infusion, and ultimately, long-term benefit from preserved myocardial function may occur. Streptokinase will be discussed further in Chapter 13.

Diazepam (Valium). Diazepam is one of a multitude of premedication choices. Ideally, the patient should be relaxed but cooperative. Patients who have high anxiety levels or low pain thresholds may need more premedication than others. We usually augment the dosage in the laboratory rather than markedly increasing dosage before the procedure. We use diazepam because it is available parenterally as well as orally in our institution. For many years, we premedicated with secobarbital (100 mg p.o.) and also had satisfactory sedation.

Lidocaine. Lidocaine is used to decrease or eliminate extrasystoles appearing during coronary artery injection. Such beats appearing in a patient without extrasystoles in their baseline tracing should be actively treated because they are possibly ischemic in origin. Lidocaine is also utilized to quiet ventricular extra beats caused by the catheter within the chamber.

TABLE 10-1   Drugs Often Used in Coronary Angiography

Drug	Premedication or Preangiography	During or After Procedure
Atropine	0.5–1 mg IM	0.5–2.5 mg IV
Nitroglycerin	0.4–0.6 mg sublingually	0.1–0.2 mg IV or intracoronary
Heparin	50 units/kg after inserting arterial line	2000 units/liter of IV and in flush solution
Ergonovine		0.05 mg IV; wait 3 min 0.10 mg IV; wait 3 min 0.25 mg IV; wait 5 min
Streptokinase		4000 IU/min to patency 2000 IU/min to patency + 60 min
Diazepam	5–10 mg p.o.	2–5 mg IV prn
Lidocaine		50–100 mg IV bolus 1–4 mg/min IV drip

Table 10-1 lists some of the drugs used most often in angiographic studies.

Atropine. 0.5–1 mg IM one hour before procedure. As prophylaxis for vasovagal episodes. 0.5–2.5 mg IV if needed for such episodes during procedure.

Nitroglycerin. 0.4 mg sublingually before injection of contrast into coronary arteries. If not given before injection, can be used when needed to rule out spasm or to relieve angina. If parenteral dose needed, 0.1–0.2 mg IV or intracoronary when needed.

Heparin. 50 units/kg as a bolus IV *after* insertion of arterial line. 2000 units per liter of IV (runs slowly through venous line during coronary study). Also used in arterial flushing solution.

Ergonovine. Three doses can be used starting from 0.05 mg IV reaching a maximum of 0.25 mg. (Some laboratories stop at 0.1 mg.) A positive response is vessel narrowing, pain, and ECG change. A physiologic response is diffuse narrowing less than 50% without pain or ECG abnormality.

Streptokinase. 4000 IU in 2 mL of 5% dextrose per minute until patency but not longer than 100 min. With vessel opening, dose reduced to 2000 IU/min in 1 ml of 5% dextrose; maintain this for 60 min. Streptokinase dose range: 200,000–400,000 IU. (Ganz, William; Swan, H.J.C.; et al.: Intracoronary thrombolysis in evolving myocardial infarction. *American Heart Journal* 101(1):4–13, 1981.)

Diazepam (Valium). 5–10 mg orally one hour before procedure. If additional sedation needed, 2–5 mg can be given IV during the procedure.

Lidocaine. Extrasystoles occurring *during* coronary artery injection should be treated with lidocaine bolus or drip. Also, ventricular catheters often cause irritability and multiple extra beats during ventriculogram. An IV bolus before injection can be used if repositioning cannot find a quiet position.

CHAPTER 11

Complications

In 1976, I wrote an article on complications that had occurred in our laboratory during the early years of our work with coronary angiography. Reviewing that article has impressed on me how far we have come since then by learning better technique and by understanding what we were doing wrong. Now, major complications occur less than 0.5% of the time. I can honestly say that the procedure has become so safe that we are now surprised if we have any complications and can rarely find obvious causes for them.

My discussion will not include all possible complications, but I will discuss those most often seen. Complications can be divided into major and minor categories. In our laboratory, we also record late complications (Table 11-1).

TABLE 11-1   Complications

Major Complications	Minor Complications	Late Complications
Myocardial infarction	Hematoma at puncture site	Renal failure
Cerebral embolus	Minor arrhythmia	Ventricular dysfunction
Peripheral arterial thrombosis	Vasovagal reaction	Late myocardial infarct
Cardiac arrest	Contrast allergy	

MAJOR COMPLICATIONS

Myocardial Infarction

In the early days, myocardial infarction was often caused by material carried on the catheter tip during the change from one catheter to another. Though the procedure of coronary arteriography has not changed much, this complication has almost disappeared. One reason may be that initial catheter flushing and contrast filling are in the descending thoracic aorta rather than in the ascending aorta, as they were in earlier days. Also, we now routinely anticoagulate with heparin throughout the procedure. Another possible reason is the improvement in the catheter material, which may collect less of the blood contents. Whatever the reason, the myocardial infarction rate in our laboratory is less than 0.5%, and I suspect this rate is similar to that of most busy catheter laboratories across the country. The most important point is careful and energetic flushing of each new catheter in the descending thoracic aorta before advancing anywhere near the cerebral or coronary arteries.

Other potential causes of myocardial infarction are air emboli down the coronary artery, which should not happen with careful technique, if your syringes are checked routinely for air, and if the syringe barrel is kept higher than the tip during injection. I believe air gets into the catheter when the syringe is filled with contrast. If the syringe is fully evacuated during the injection, a small amount of air ends up in the catheter. Because you do not draw back into the syringe before each injection, the air is infected with the next contrast bolus. This is a relatively rare problem and should not occur if care is used in drawing up contrast.

Myocardial infarction may also occur when thrombus or plaque is dislodged by a guide wire or catheter tip entering the vessel orifice. Guide wires should be prevented from entering the coronary arteries, since they can not only dislodge material but can also injure or puncture the vessel wall. Catheter entry, of course, is necessary and if this is the source of the dislodgement, it cannot be prevented. Also, if a catheter blocks a vessel and stops blood flow, ischemia and the potential for an infarct exist. This problem should never occur if pressure is monitored through the catheter end hole, since obstruction should immediately be noted if pressure damps, and catheter withdrawal would allow flow to resume. Finally, myocardial infarctions have occurred due to vessel spasm. In patients with atypical or Prinzmetal angina, spontaneous spasm or artificially induced spasm has occasionally caused a myocardial infarction. This problem can usually be avoided by prompt use of nitroglycerin.

The most common cause of infarction, however, is the entrance of solid blood products into the coronary artery. This often occurs during catheter exchange.

Catheter insertion by the percutaneous technique is usually performed as follows: After the needle puncture of the artery, a guide wire is introduced into the artery through the needle lumen. This wire is like a guitar string but is often coated with Teflon. After insertion of the wire, the needle is slid off the end of the wire and a catheter is threaded over the wire and inserted into the vessel. The catheter tip is tapered to be a tight fit over the wire for easy entry into the artery. Of course, the wire must be longer than the catheter so that it can be removed once the catheter is inserted. If a different catheter is to be inserted after that catheter has been used, the guide wire is once again inserted through the catheter tip into the vessel lumen. The first catheter is then removed and a second catheter inserted in the manner just described. Here is where the myocardial complication is set in motion. Because the first catheter has been in the bloodstream, fibrin can accumulate on the catheter's outer wall. When this catheter is removed, the fibrin is wiped off, but will remain on the guide wire just where the wire enters the femoral artery lumen. When the new catheter is inserted, the fibrin may be picked up on the catheter tip, and as the catheter is advanced, the fibrin may be injected inadvertently into a coronary artery or possibly a cerebral vessel. As mentioned previously, catheter exchange and energetic flushing in the descending aorta, with the addition of heparinization, should minimize this complication.

Cerebral Embolus

Cerebral embolus is also rare but, like a myocardial infarction, may have disastrous aftereffects. The complication is similar to a myocardial infarction in that foreign material injected from within the catheter reaches a cerebral location or a catheter or guide wire dislodges material into the cerebral vessels. The symptoms that follow relate to the area of the brain affected. Though the effects are often temporary, neurologic defects occasionally persist. Prevention again involves careful flushing of catheters and caution with catheter and guide wire manipulation in the area of the cerebral vessels.

Peripheral Arterial Thrombosis

Coronary arteriography can be performed by the brachial approach through a surgical cutdown on the brachial artery or by a percutaneous approach from the femoral artery or, occasionally, the axillary artery. Thrombosis following brachial artery closure is fairly uncommon when the procedure is performed by skilled hands, but it does occur. The more common causes of thrombosis relate to unskilled closure of the arteriotomy, with the formation of intimal flaps that form a nidus for thrombosis, or closure without evidence of good blood flow from both proximal and distal arterial segments. If good pulsation is not available after closure, reexploration should be considered before the patient leaves the catheterization laboratory.

Percutaneous techniques, though relatively traumatic to the vessel wall, will rarely be followed by thrombosis if this major point is kept in mind: *You need not obstruct blood flow to get hemostasis at the puncture site.* The total obstruction of the vessel during compression is the forerunner of the thrombosis. If you can feel a downstream pulse while you are compressing the vessel, you will rarely lose the femoral pulse. This technique is so successful that we routinely monitor the level of pressure on the femoral artery by palpating the dorsalis pedis pulse simultaneously. The correct pressure level is one that controls bleeding but also allows palpation of a distal pulse. In addition, you will often feel a bruit during correct pressure application, and this evidence of flow while the vessel is compressed almost guarantees absence of thrombosis at the entry site. Although there are always exceptions, I have only seen pulse loss when there was occlusion of the vessel during compression. Also, I have not seen a patient leave our laboratory with a good pulse only to have that pulse disappear after the patient returns to bed. Instead, I have seen the opposite—a return to a good pulse when a patient has left our laboratory with an absent or diminished pulse. However, we do not wait very long for this to happen, and if there are peripheral signs related to a decreased blood flow, we have the surgeons explore the vessel and reconstitute good flow.

This complication, though common in the early years of our practice, has virtually disappeared with good compression techniques. A special note of caution must be raised about axillary artery punctures. Although the compression technique is essentially the same, you must be very cautious. If there are peripheral symptoms, such as parasthesia or strength loss following this procedure, they are indications for exploration even though a good pulse exists because a small amount of blood compressing adjacent nerve roots can cause severe neurologic deficits. A final comment relates to the virtual absence of peripheral embolic symptoms during the removal or changing of catheters. One would imagine that some material on the catheter would proceed distally and create problems. Whether natural anticoagulation or the lack of such particles on the catheter eliminates this complication is unclear. Again, it is a phenomenon that does not seem to occur. I am not sure whether anticoagulation, particle size, or collateral vessels prevent it.

Cardiac Arrest (Ventricular Fibrillation)

Most often, cardiac arrest is due to ventricular fibrillation, often following bradycardia. Mild bradycardia occurs routinely after each coronary injection; however, for some reason, occasionally the bradycardia is prolonged and progresses to ventricular fibrillation. Because catheterization rooms are equipped with defibrillators, such equipment should be applied quickly and at appropriate wattage to revert the patient to his or her routine rhythm. Occasionally patients become extremely anxious after the defibrillation. Some may develop angina, and a few have significant ventricular dysfunction. Whether to continue with the study is up to the angiographer and relates to the patient's condition. In our laboratory, if we can continue the study, we do, and have not created new problems for the patient.

MINOR COMPLICATIONS

Hematoma

Hematoma can occur during the procedure if oozing occurs along the catheter or if bleeding occurs during catheter exchange because of inadequate compression. It can also occur following catheter removal if compression is not adequate over the vessel. Patients' problems are additive, particularly if the patient is obese or hypertensive. The important point is not to panic: As long as your puncture was below the inguinal ligament and you can control the pulse (again, by using the dorsalis pedis or other peripheral pulse), bleeding will usually stop.

Rarely, and often when there is no hematoma, bleeding just will not stop. If you are sure the effects of heparin have been reversed and the vessel has been compressed for a prolonged period, vessel wall laceration and repair must be considered.

Minor Arrhythmias

Occasionally, superventricular tachycardias occur. These often break spontaneously and should only be treated actively if they persist or if anginal symptoms occur. Also, catheters in the ventricle cause multiple extra beats. These can be controlled with lidocaine, if necessary.

Vasovagal Reaction

Vasovagal reaction most often occurs during initial catheter insertion or even during local anesthetic injection. The classic symptoms are bradycardia, hypotension, a pale face, and clammy skin. The treatment is to elevate the legs and administer atropine, often as much as 2–3 mg. Often, atropine alone will not make the patient feel or look better. Elevation of the legs seems to be needed as well. Also, occasionally there seems to be a vagal effect without slowing of the heart rate. In this case, though elevation of the legs often results in improvement, atropine seems also to be beneficial.

Contrast Reaction

Reaction to iodinated contrast material may vary from sneezing and itching or hives to bronchial spasm, angioneurotic edema, and vascular collapse. The simple reactions usually respond to parenteral antihistamines (Benadryl 25 mg IV). More severe reactions require epinephrine, blood pressure support, and, occasionally, intubation. Severe reactions are extraordinarily rare on arterial side injections but rather more common during venous studies.

Patients with prior contrast reactions who need angiographic study are premedicated in our laboratory with oral steroids ideally for three days before the examination and given antihistamine and IV steroids at the time of the examination. Our experience with this regimen has been good, although some feel that such treatment is of little value. Much has been written on contrast allergy, but the subject is beyond the scope of this book.

LATE COMPLICATIONS

Renal Failure

Though iodinated contrast has a deleterious effect on the kidneys, it can be used with relative safety even in patients with some depression of renal function. The important point is to keep the patient *well hydrated.* Do not withhold oral fluids unless you plan to infuse intravenous fluid before study. Nursing units are accustomed to npo orders before catheterization laboratory studies, so even if you order fluids by mouth, be sure the patient has received *and* ingested them. It now seems that renal dysfunction may not relate to contrast overload (3–4 mL/kg is routine) but rather to dehydration before the procedure. Although renal dysfunction does occur, the abnormality usually reverts spontaneously. In some patients, hemodialysis has been required.

Ventricular Dysfunction

Some patients, particularly older ones with multivessel disease and poor ventricular function, seem to deteriorate rapidly after a coronary arteriogram. Whether this is caused by the stress of the procedure, disturbance of a precarious balance, or chemical effects of the contrast material involved is unknown. But rarely, following this procedure, such patients will slowly deteriorate and die in the hospital. It is difficult to predict this likelihood beforehand, but patients whose disease is far advanced and who have multiple system failure seem to be prime candidates.

Late Myocardial Infarction

Occasionally, patients return to the floor and have a myocardial infarction within 24 hours of the procedure. This is considered a complication in many laboratories, though obviously the infarct occurs in patients who have angina and who are at risk any time. Even though one could argue the validity of considering such late infarcts to be complications of the arteriographic study, they are considered complications in most laboratories.

In summary, this chapter does not include all possible complications, but only those most often seen. As noted, complications are uncommon (major complications occur in less than 0.5% of studies), but they do occur occasionally.

CHAPTER 12

Generating a Report

In reporting coronary arteriography, as in all radiographic angiography reports, we start routinely with a short clinical history. This is followed by a technical paragraph, including the type and size of the catheters, the volume of contrast, and the position of the heart during the ventriculogram. The technical description includes any problems with the study, such as unusual anatomy, difficulty in catheter placement, or complications. The information is designed to be helpful if a repeat study needs to be performed.

The final part of the report is descriptive, detailing the angiographic findings. In our reports we describe the vessels first, then the ventriculogram. The vessels are described separately, each vessel described proximally to distally. The order of the report is as follows:

1. Dominance
2. *Left coronary artery*
   Left main coronary artery
   LAD
   Diagonals
3. *Left circumflex artery*
   Marginals
4. *Right coronary artery*
   Marginals

The inferior wall vessels are described under either the left circumflex or right coronary, depending on dominance. A language has been developed to describe degrees of severity, states of the distal vessel, and morphology of lesions. This process has been necessary to transmit interpretive information to nonviewers so that they can act medically or surgically. The trick to developing a good language is to be sure it is reproducible by varying groups of viewers, understood by different coronary angiographers, and satisfactory in its simplicity in that the language is not more sophisticated than it needs to be.

Before moving on, try the exercise in Figure 12-1. (The number of vessels to identify keeps increasing as we progress through this book, but the nomenclature remains descriptive.) Figure 12-1 lists a number of vessels or vessel segments. Try going through them and filling in as many names as you can. The answers are in the answer key on page 94.

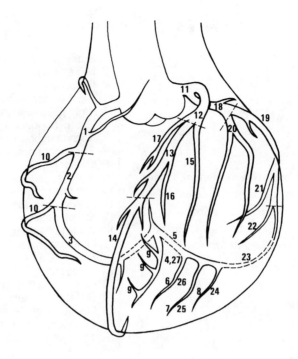

FIGURE 12-1.

1. _____   15. _____
2. _____   16. _____
3. _____   17. _____
4. _____   18. _____
5. _____   19. _____
6. _____   20. _____
7. _____   21. _____
8. _____   22. _____
9. _____   23. _____
10. _____   24. _____
11. _____   25. _____
12. _____   26. _____
13. _____   27. _____
14. _____

The vessels are described as follows:

1. Normal
2. Single discrete lesion
3. Multiple discrete lesions
4. Discrete aneurysmal
5. Multiple aneurysmal
6. Diffuse disease
7. Tubular

As mentioned previously, loss of lumen is described as percent of cross-sectional diameter loss.

Also included in the vessel description is an evaluation of the remainder of the vessel. The purpose of this is to allow assessment for bypass. This is the terminology that we use:

Normal size, not diseased
Normal size, diseased
Small size, not diseased
Small size, diseased
Poorly visualized
Not visible

After the vessels are discussed, the ventriculogram is described, again, fairly concisely. The description is along the lines mentioned in Chapter 5 and includes segmental motion, chamber size, contractility, chamber contents, wall thickness, and valve motion.

The final part of the report is your overall impression, including whether disease exists, its severity, and some comment on the overall condition of the ventricles.

ANSWER KEY
1. Proximal right coronary
2. Midright coronary
3. Distal right coronary
4. Right posterior descending*
5. Right posterolateral*
6. First right posterolateral*
7. Second right posterolateral*
8. Third right posterolateral*
9. Inferior septal
10. Right (acute) marginals
11. Left main coronary
12. Proximal left anterior descending
13. Midleft anterior descending
14. Distal left anterior descending
15. First diagonal
16. Second diagonal
17. First septal
18. Proximal circumflex
19. Distal circumflex
20. First left (obtuse) marginal
21. Second left (obtuse) marginal
22. Third left (obtuse) marginal
23. Left AV
24. First left posterolateral*
25. Second left posterolateral*
26. Third left posterolateral*
27. Left posterior descending*

*Note that right or left designation depends on dominance.

CHAPTER 13

New Techniques

I have tried to stay with basic concepts throughout this primer; however, several new procedures have become so useful in the diagnosis and treatment of coronary heart disease that it is really necessary to explain these advances. Let me emphasize that the information should be considered a "broad brush" and that those of you who are interested in applying such procedures to practice must pursue these subjects by reviewing what is happening at the time you plan to do such procedures. These techniques change and are modified often as they are tried and tested by many angiographers on many patients. Therefore, many changes and improvements will probably occur within a short time.

PERCUTANEOUS TRANSLUMINAL ANGIOPLASTY

The aortocoronary saphenous vein bypass operation is very satisfactory as the current surgical procedure to relieve angina. Though the results have been excellent, you must not forget the extent of the surgical procedure. The surgery requires sternal splitting and major intrathoracic surgery. Also to be considered are the veins utilized for the procedure; these must be removed from the patient's thighs. The procedure necessitates about 7–10 days in the hospital, and charges for such a procedure run between $10,000 and $20,000. Therefore, there are several reasons to find quicker, less traumatic, and less expensive methods of treating coronary artery narrowings.

Development of the Procedure

A nonoperative approach to vascular occlusive disease was developed in 1964 by Dotter and Judkins and was successfully used for peripheral atherosclerotic vascular narrowings. Their original system used a series of coaxial catheters, and by passing these catheters of increasing size over one another, they gradually dilated a narrowed area. Although a vessel could not be dilated back to its original luminal diameter, even slight improvement often greatly alleviated symptoms. Remember from a previous discussion of flow down a narrowed vessel that even small improvements in radius have great effect on area and thus on flow. However, though this system was effective in selective cases, the method never became popular, and surgery for occlusive vascular disease remained the standard.

In 1974, Grüntzig and Hopff developed a flexible double-lumen balloon catheter, and that development has caused nonoperative treatment of vascular narrowings to emerge as a viable and important procedure. The balloon is made of polyvinyl chloride and can be inflated up to 6 atmospheres of pressure. These catheters inflate to a precisely predetermined diameter and are available in varying sizes. The balloons can be inserted percutaneously; because they are so flexible, they can be manipulated into almost any vessel. It is this flexibility that has allowed a procedure initially designed for peripheral vessels to be used in the coronary arteries.

Current Technique

Coronary transluminal angioplasty requires modification of the peripheral arterial technique. Figure 13–1 shows the steps in the procedure. Instead of direct insertion of the balloon catheter into the artery, a guiding catheter is used to ease placement into the coronary vessels. The guiding catheter is designed similarly to coronary catheters, but the end is not tapered. It is inserted percutaneously and advanced into the coronary artery of choice.

The balloon catheter is then inserted into the coronary artery through the guiding catheter. Radiopaque markers on the balloon catheter mark the proximal and distal ends of the balloon. This allows correct placement of the balloon in relationship to the coronary artery narrowing that is to be dilated. The balloon is then inflated using a contrast-containing solution that allows visualization of the balloon. The balloon is dilated to 4–5 atmospheres for 4–5 seconds at a time. Blood flow is maintained to the distal vessel between injections, but during the short dilatation period there is no flow distally. This has not been associated with complications.

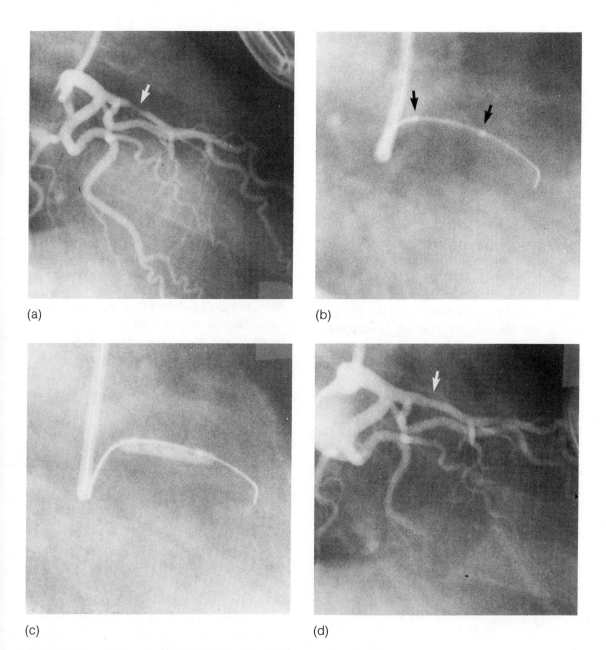

(a)

(b)

(c)

(d)

FIGURE 13-1. a: RAO projection with injection of the left coronary artery. An 80% symmetric stenosis of the proximal left anterior descending artery is noted (arrow). b: Guiding catheter and balloon catheter in place in proximal LAD. Radio-opaque markers identify balloon position (arrowheads). c: Balloon catheter inflated with contrast-containing solution. Note smooth wall suggesting full compression of plaque. d: Postdilatation angiogram in RAO projection showing improvement in the area of prior narrowing (arrow).

There are several signs that the procedure has been successful. Often, as the balloon is inflated to its full diameter, a deformity in the contrast-filled balloon is produced by the vessel narrowing. That is the importance of seeing the balloon, since with continued inflations these deformities disappear, signaling full compression of the stenosis. Also, as pressure can be simultaneously monitored through the guiding catheter and the balloon catheter, a previously measured gradient often disappears after several balloon inflations.

The procedure is dramatic when successful and certainly is a welcome alternative to surgery. It is quicker, less traumatic, and much less expensive. The results at present reveal about a 10% restenosis rate, most often occurring in the first six months. Redilatation is routine, and the results of the second dilatation are often better than those of the first. Although initial patient selection leaned toward the easier, more proximal lesions, present practice now includes dilatation of more difficult distal ones as well as treatment of lesions in several vessels during a single procedure. The major complication is converting a high-grade lesion to total obstruction at the time of dilatation. This occurrence requires immediate surgical intervention. Depending on operator skill and patient selection, the likelihood of the complication is 4%–10%.

STREPTOKINASE INFUSION TO DISSOLVE INTRACORONARY THROMBUS

The concept of an agent to dissolve clots has always been attractive. This has been true for clots of the deep venous system and the peripheral or pulmonary arterial trees. But there is no comparison as to how important it would be if coronary arterial thrombus could be dissolved. The importance relates to more than the potential avoidance of surgery if the clot were dissolved. It relates more directly to preserving heart muscle that is lost very early in the postinfarct period. That muscle preservation is what defines long-term survival after infarct, as well as quality of life.

Heparin has been used for many years to prevent pulmonary thromboembolism, deep venous thrombus, and emboli following valve surgery. Though effective in those clinical situations, heparin has not been directly used to dissolve clots within the coronary vascular system. Streptokinase has emerged as the agent that has been successful in achieving that goal.

Streptokinase was discovered in 1933, when it was observed that a filtrate of group C beta-hemolytic streptococci lysed human plasma clot. Subsequent studies show that an activator substance acted on plasminogen to produce and activate the enzyme plasmin. The activator was named streptokinase. Streptokinase has been used extensively for acute arterial occlusions. Varying doses have been used, and it has been administered from intravenous and intraarterial sites. Many combinations of dose and site have produced successful results. Some of the early experience was in the hands of Ganz and Rentrop, who infused streptokinase into the coronary artery through the coronary catheter or through a smaller catheter advanced up against

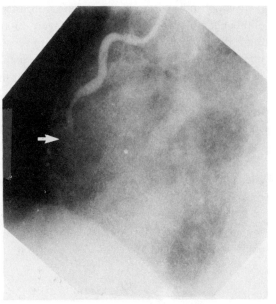
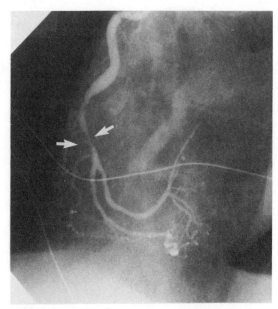

(a)   (b)

FIGURE 13-2. Example of a streptokinase infusion. On the left (a) is the right coronary artery injection in the LAO projection. Total obstruction is seen in the mid portion of the vessel. (arrow) On the right (b) is the vessel 90 minutes after streptokinase infusion. The area of narrowing where the thrombosis and obstruction occurred can be seen (arrows). The distal right vessel can be clearly seen, is dominant, and is essentially normal.

the clot. These studies showed the potential success of such a procedure, and in most of their patients, the occluded vessel opened (Figure 13-2).

Since this initial experience, streptokinase infusion has become a useful, and in some practices routine, procedure if the patient reaches the hospital early enough. Speed in reaching the laboratory is crucial if myocardium is to be preserved—the major goal of this effort. Note that myocardial salvage does not always occur. There may be partial or no recovery even though the infusion was timely.

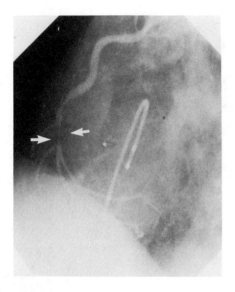

(a)

It is not unusual to see streptokinase infusion and balloon dilatation used together (Figure 13-3). Since thrombus usually gathers at an area of vessel narrowing, dissolution of the thrombus does nothing for the preexisting narrowing. It is natural to assume that rethrombosis can occur if nothing further is done about the narrowing. The procedure of choice obviously depends on a variety of issues, but one of them is whether the vessel can be reached for dilatation. If not, surgery would be the only choice. Balloon dilatation has emerged as a successful and increasingly used treatment.

It is useful to pause a moment and consider the events that have affected this patient whose angiograms are shown in Figures 13-2 and 13-3. In

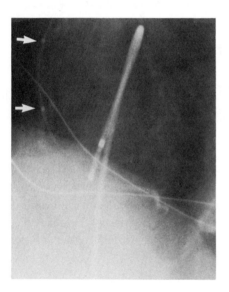

(b)   (c)

FIGURE 13-3. Example of a balloon dilatation of the same patient several days later. In b the balloon is in place as noted by the marker positions (arrows). In c, the postdilatation angiogram is seen. Note the wide dilatation of the previously narrowed segment (arrows). Also note the spasm of the a portion of the vessel just distal to the dilated segment (curved arrow).

the past he would have had chest pain, entered the coronary care unit, and probably have gone home to recover from his infarction. It is likely that he would have lost considerable inferior wall myocardium. If pain had persisted, he would have returned to the hospital for an evaluation that would eventually lead to surgery. Even if surgery were successful, the myocardium could have been lost. Shortly after admission, this patient had streptokinase infusion, which opened the vessel and preserved his myocardium. Three days later the vessel was dilated, eliminating the need for surgery. These are two important improvements in the care of the coronary patient.

DIGITAL SUBTRACTION ANGIOGRAPHY

Digital subtraction angiography is an imaging technique that has become exceedingly popular, primarily because it allows good visualization of arterial vessels following contrast injection on the venous side of the vascular system. This is possible because of image enhancement techniques inherent with this system. The outcome is that many patients can have vascular procedures as outpatients and need not go through the inconvenience and expense of hospitalization. Successful visualization of the extracranial carotid system has been of particular value because of clinical signs and symptoms from that anatomic area in an increasingly aged population. The ability to study that vascular tree without inserting catheters selectively obviously eliminates procedural problems in an at-risk population. As the quality and versatility of this type of imaging have improved, routine abdominal as well as femoral vascular studies are also performed.

The technique uses a fluoroscopic system that allows enhancement of an image by removing unwanted parts of the same image. The unwanted portions are "subtracted." For example, bones and soft tissues can be eliminated from an image, allowing better visualization of vessels. This is accomplished in a fashion similar to subtraction techniques that have been used in radiology departments for years. As part of a contrast filming series, a film is taken before the contrast is injected. This film, which is identical to the series of film that follows, only differs in that no contrast has reached the vascular tree. If this first film is copied in a reversal mode (whites become blacks) and then superimposed on the contrast-containing film of interest, a final film copy of the two-film overlay will show only the contrast-filled areas—the only areas of difference between the mask and the contrast film. The technique allows subtraction of the common areas.

Digital subtraction techniques differ in several ways, but conceptually the methods are similar. In the digital mode, a fluoroscopic image is used rather than a radiograph. For a contrast study that is to be performed on fluoroscopy, viewing is started before contrast injection. A frame before contrast reaches the vascular area is again used as a mask. This masking frame can be used to subtract any of the subsequent images that follow.

Although similar to cut film subtraction, digital subtraction digitizes the image from the TV camera image of the output phosphor of the image intensifier. The digital image is stored as a matrix with varying numbers of pixels (picture elements). Since the image is viewed on a cathode ray tube (CRT), one can enhance various parts of the image electronically, as well as being able to subtract.

New equipment allows production of 30 frames in a 1 second period. For cardiac studies, an increased framing speed was necessary to visualize cardiac motion and vessel filling. In Figure 13–4 are images of coronary arterial injections. These have been produced on the arterial side rather than the venous. Although this seems at variance with the stated objective of avoiding arterial puncture and hospital admission by using a venous injection, another important benefit of digital subtraction angiography is realized. This relates to the decreased amount of contrast needed for these examinations. This is particularly important in patients with cardiovascular problems because it is not unusual for this patient group to have vascular abnormalities in the peripheral and cerebral vessels as well. Multiple diagnostic studies during one examination have been hazardous because of the contrast volume and its effect on patients having abnormal renal function. Digital studies allow safe study of all these systems during one admission.

In Figures 13-4a and b you will recognize the left coronary artery injection in the LAO and RAO projections. Figures 13-4c and d are similar projections of the right coronary artery. Note the quality of films obtained. Since digital units are often in a C-arm configuration, all of the angled views could be obtained.

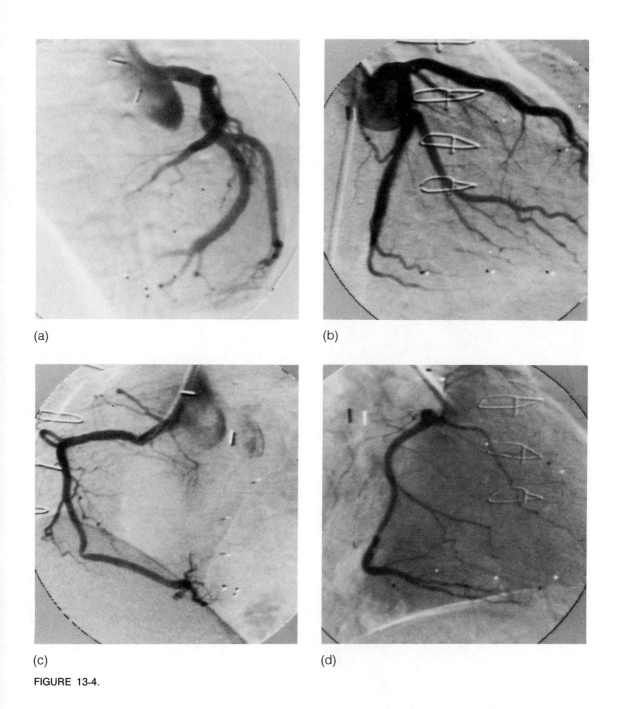

(a)

(b)

(c)

(d)

FIGURE 13-4.

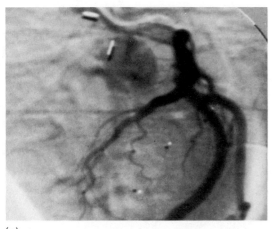

(a)

Figure 13-5 shows three presentations of the LAO left coronary artery injection, but each one is enhanced somewhat differently. Note the difference in background between the frames as well as the presentation of the vascular structures. This ability to enhance is a benefit of digitizing and of being able to display the information in different forms. Digital filming will surely become a routine function in radiology departments. Its use for cardiac studies will probably continue to expand.

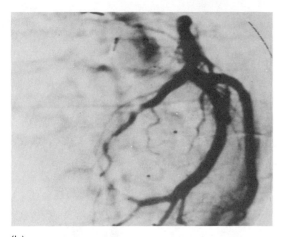

(b)

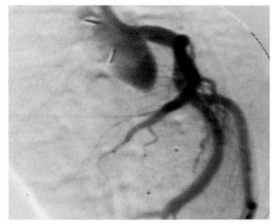

(c)

FIGURE 13-5.

CHAPTER 1

Abrams, H.L. 1961. *Angiography*, 2nd ed. Vol. 1. Boston: Little, Brown & Co.

Abrams, H.L., and Adams, D.F. 1969. The coronary angiogram: structural and functional aspects. *N. Engl. J. Med.* 281:1276–1285.

Adams, D.F.; Abrams, H.L.; and Rutler, M. 1972. The roentgen and pathology of coronary artery disease. *Semin. Roentgenol.* 7:319.

Davies, M.D. 1970. Cardiac roentgenology: the loop and circle approach. *Radiology* 95:157–160.

Margolis, J.R.; Chen, J.T.T.; Kong, Y.; et al. 1980. The diagnostic and prognostic significance of coronary artery calcification. *Radiology* 137:609–616.

CHAPTER 3

Cipriano, P.R.; Sacks, A.H.; and Reitz, B.A. 1980. The effect of stenosis of bypass grafts on coronary blood flow: a mechanical model study. *Circulation* 62(1):61–66.

Chaitman, B.R.; Fisher, L.D.; Bourassa, M.G.; et al. 1981. Effect of coronary bypass surgery on survival patterns in subsets of patients with left main coronary artery disease: report of the Collaborative Study in Coronary Artery Surgery (CASS). *Am. J. Cardiol.* 48:765–777.

Conley, N.J.; Ely, R.L.; Kisslo, J.; et al. 1978. The prognostic spectrum of left main stenosis. *Circulation* 57:947–952.

Feldman, R.L.; Nichols, W.W.; Pepine, C.J.; and Conti, C.R. 1978. Hemodynamic significance of the length of a coronary arterial narrowing. *Am. J. Cardiol.* 41:865–871.

Gould, K.L.; Lipscomb K.; and Hamilton, G.W. 1974. Physiologic basis for assessing critical coronary stenosis: instantaneous flow response and regional distribution during coronary hyperemia as measures of coronary flow reserve. *Cardiol.* 33:87–94.

Gould, K.L.; Lipscomb, K.; and Calvert, C. 1975. Compensatory changes of the distal coronary vascular bed during progressive coronary constriction. *Circulation* 51:1085–1094.

Levin, D.C.; Beckmann, C.F. and Serur, J.R. 1980. Vascular resistance changes distal to progressive arterial stenosis: a critical re-evaluation of the concept of vasodilator reserve. *Invest. Radiol.* 15:120–128.

May, A.G.; Van de Berg, L.; DeWeese, J.A.; and Rob, C.G. 1963. Critical arterial stenosis. *Surgery* 54(1):250–258.

Santamore, W.P., and Walinsky, P. 1980. Altered coronary flow responses to vasoactive drugs in the presence of coronary arterial stenosis in the dog. *Am. J. Cardiol.* 45:276–285.

Schuster, E.H.; Griffith, L.S.; and Bulkley, B.H. 1981. Preponderance of acute proximal left anterior descending coronary arterial lesions in fatal myocardial infarction: a clinicopathologic study. *Am. J. Cardiol.* 47(6):1189–1196.

Selzer, A. 1980. Strategy for treatment of left main coronary artery disease. *Am. J. Cardiol.* 46: 517.

Stone, P.H., and Goldschlager, N. 1979. Left main coronary artery disease: review and appraisal. *Cardiovasc. Med.* 4:165–178.

CHAPTER 4

Bunnell. I.L.; Greene, D.G.; et al. 1973. The half-axial projection: a new look at the proximal left coronary artery. *Circulation* 18:1151.

Eldh, P., and Silverman, J.F. 1974. Methods of studying the proximal left anterior descending coronary artery. *Radiology* 113:738–740.

Elliott, L.P.; Bream, P.R.; Soto, B.; et al. 1981. Significance of the caudal left-anterior-oblique view in analyzing the left main coronary artery and its major branches. *Radiology* 139:39–43.

Grainger, R.G. 1981. Terminology for radiographic projections. *Br.Heart J.* 45:109–111.

Miller, R.A.; Warkentin, D.L.; Felix, W.G.; et al. 1980. Angulated views in coronary angiography. *Am. J. Radiol.* 134:407–412.

CHAPTER 5

Cohn, P.F.; Maddox, D.E.; Holman, B.L.; and See, J.R. 1980. Effect of coronary collateral vessels on regional myocardial blood flow in patients with coronary artery disease. *Am. J. Cardiol.* 46:359–364.

Goldstein, R.E.; Stinson, E.B.; Scherer, J.L.; et al. 1974. Intraoperative coronary collateral function in patients with coronary occlusive disease. *Circulation* 49:298–308.

Levin, D.C. 1974. Pathways and functional significance of the coronary collateral circulation. *Circulation* 50:831.

Levin, D.C.; Beckmann, C.F.; Sos, T.A.; and Sniderman, K. 1981. The effect of coronary artery bypass on collateral circulation. *Radiology* 141:317–322.

CHAPTER 6

Wolf, N.M.; Kreulen, T.H.; Bove, A.A.; et al. 1978. Left ventricular function following coronary bypass surgery. *Circulation* 58(1):63–70.

CHAPTER 9

Amplatz, K.; Formanek, C.; Stanger, P.; and Wilson, W. 1967. Mechanics of selective coronary artery catheterization via femoral approach. *Radiology* 89:1040–1047.

Brasch, C. 1980. Allergic reactions to contrast media: accumulated evidence. *Am. J. Radiol.* 134:797–801.

Conti, R.C. 1977. Reviews of contemporary laboratory methods: coronary arteriography. *Circulation* 55:(2):227–237.

El Gamal, M.; Slegers, L.; Bonnier, H.; et al. 1980. Selective coronary arteriography with a preformed single catheter: percutaneous femoral technique. *Am. J. Radiol.* 135:630–632.

Judkins, M.P., 1967. Selective coronary arteriograph—a percutaneous transfemoral technique. *Radiology* 89:815.

CHAPTER 10

Conti, R.C. 1977. Reviews of contemporary laboratory methods: coronary arteriography. *Circulation* 55(2):227–237.

Mulcahy, R.; Daly, L.; Graham, I.; et al. 1981. Unstable angina: natural history and determinants of prognosis. *Am. J. Cardiol.* 48:525–528.

CHAPTER 11

Meany, T.F.; Lalli, A.F.; and Alfidi, R.J. 1973. *Complications and legal implications of radiologic special procedures.* St. Louis: The C. V. Mosby Co.

CHAPTER 13

Block, P.C.; Myler, R.K.; Stertzer, S.; and Fallow, J.T. 1981. Morphology after transluminal angioplasty in human beings. *N. Engl. J. Med.* 305(7):382–385.

Crummy, A.B.; Stieghorst, M.F.; Turski, P.A.; et al. 1982. Digital subtraction angiography: current status and use of intra-arterial injection. *Radiology* 145:303–307.

Dotter, C.T., and Judkins, M.P. 1964. Transluminal treatment of arteriosclerotic obstruction. Description of a new technic and a preliminary report of its application. *Circulation* 30:654–670.

Ganz, W.; Buchbinder, N.; Marcus, H.; et al. 1981. Intracoronary thrombolysis in evolving myocardial infarction. *Clin. Invest.* 101(1):4–13.

Grüntzig, A., and Hopff, H. 1974. Perkutane Rekanalisation chronischer arterieller Verschlüsse mit einem neuen Dilatationskatheter. Modifikation der Dotter-Technik. *Dtsch. Med. Wochenschr.* 99:2502–2505, 2511 (Ger.).

Kent, K.M.; Bonow, R.O.; Rosing, D.R.; et al. 1982. Improved myocardial function during exercise after successful percutaneous transluminal coronary angioplasty. *N. Engl. J. Med.* 306:441–446.

Levy, J.M.; Hessel, S.J.; Nykamp, P.W.; et al. 1982. Digital subtraction angiography; the community hospital experience. *Diagnostic Imaging* 4(3):23–28.

Markis, J.E.; Malagold, M.; Parker, J.A.; et al. 1981. Myocardial salvage after intracoronary thrombolysis with streptokinase in acute myocardial infarction. *N. Engl. J. Med.* 305:777.

Mistretta, C.A. 1982. Digital subtraction angiography: the shape of things to come. *Diagnostic Imaging* 4(11):36–40.

Rentrop, P.; Blanke, H.; Karsch, K.R.; et al. 1981. Selective intracoronary thrombolysis in acute myocardial infarction and unstable angina pectois. *Circulation* 63:307–317.

Sharma, G.V.R.K.; Cella, G.; Parisi, A.F.; and Sasahara, A.A. 1982. Thrombolytic therapy. In *Drug therapy*, editor J. Koch-Weser. *N. Engl. J. Med.* 306(21): 1268–1276.

Sobel, B.E. In press. Coronary thrombolysis: some unresolved issues. *Am. J. Med.*

Tegtmeyer, C.J. 1983. Balloon angioplasty: putting catheters to work in place of the scalpel. *Diagnostic Imaging* 5(4):40–49.

van Breda, A. 1982. Regional thrombolysis in the treatment of peripheral arterial occlusions. *Appl. Radiol.* 2(4):63–71.

This section is designed to give you a little extra practice in identifying the segments and estimating the percentages of luminal loss. Just mark the percentages and vessel names in the drawings provided on the right pages; answers, and some additional information about each case, are given on the left pages.

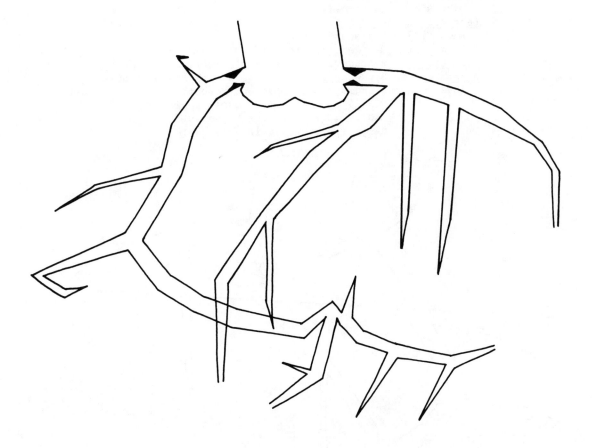

QUIZ #1.   CORONARY ARTERIOGRAPHY

<u>Anatomy of native coronary arteries:</u>
  Dominance: Right
  LAD branches: Diag 1.....small
                Dist LAD...medium
  Cx branches: Intermed...medium
                ObMarg 1....medium
                Dist Cx......small

<u>Right Coronary Artery:</u>
  Prox RCA ...95% discrete stenosis
  Mid RCA ....is normal
  Dist RCA ...is normal

<u>Left Main Coronary Artery:</u>
  LMCA .....95% discarete stenosis

<u>Left Anterior Descending:</u> Normal
<u>Left Circumflex Artery:</u> Normal
<u>Assessment of Bypassability</u> of vessels with lesions 50%
   (based on the angiographic size and morphology of the distal vessel)
          RCA.................is bypassabale
          LAD.................is bypassable
          Cx..................is bypassable

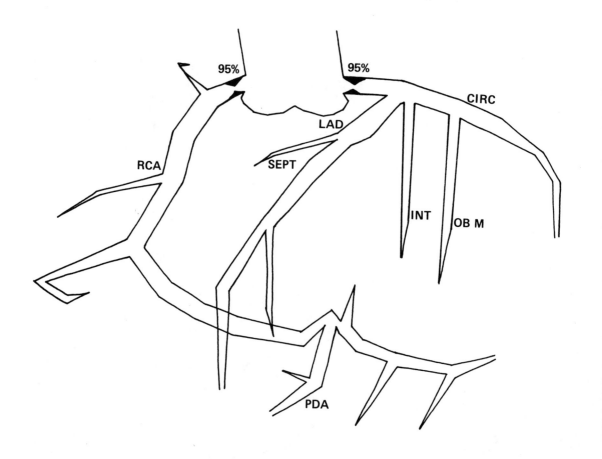

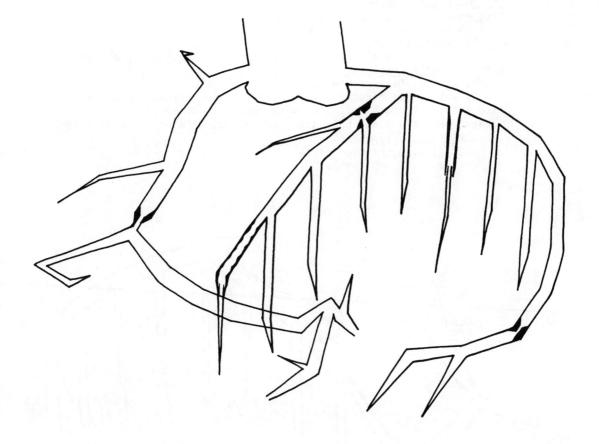

QUIZ #2.   <u>CORONARY ARTERIOGRAPHY</u>
            <u>Anatomy of native coronary arteries:</u>
              Dominance: Mixed
              LAD branches: Diag 1....small   Diag 2 medium... Diag 3....medium
                             Dist LAD..medium
              Cx branches: Intermed ..small
                             ObMarg 1..medium   ObMarg 2..small   ObMarg 3..medium
                             Dist Cx...large
            <u>Right Coronary Artery:</u>
              Mid RCA....85% discrete stenosis; distal to lesion, segment small
              Dist RCA...is normal
            <u>Left Main Coronary Artery</u>: Normal
            <u>Left Anterior Descending:</u>
               Prox LAD...80% discrete stenosis
               Mid LAD....is normal
               Dist LAD....40% diffuse disease; distal to lesion, segment small
            <u>Left Circumflex Artery:</u>
               Dist Cx ....75% discrete stenosis
               ObMarg 1....30% tubular stenosis; distal to lesion, segment small
            Assessment of Bypassability of vessels with lesions 50%
               (based on the angiographic size and morphology of the distal vessel)
                 RCA.......is bypassable
                 LAD.......is not bypassable
                 Cx........is bypassable

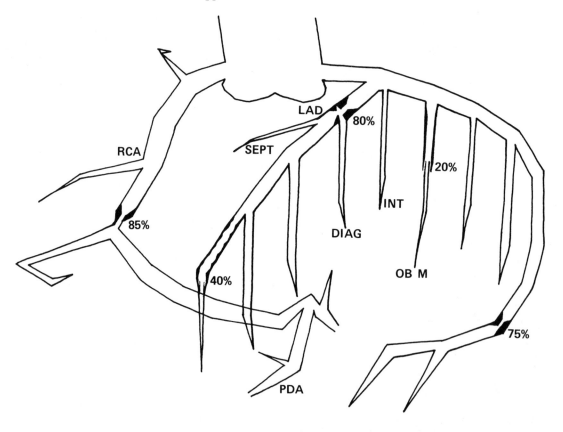

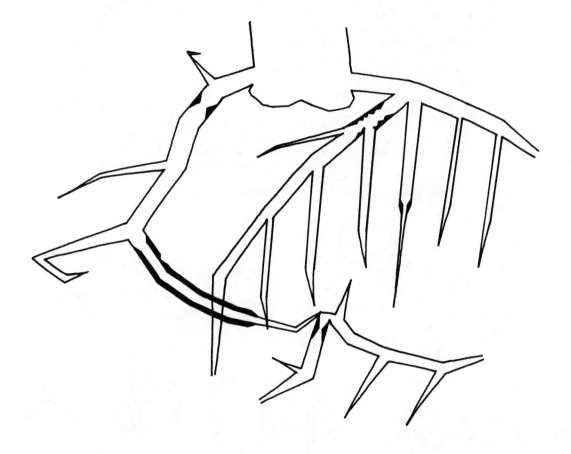

QUIZ #3.   CORONARY ARTERIOGRAPHY

<u>Anatomy of native coronary arteries</u>

  Dominance: Right

  LAD branches: Diag 1...medium   Diag 2...medium   Diag 3....small
                  Dist LAD..medium

  Cx branches: Intermed..large
                  ObMarg 1..small   ObMarg 2..small
                  Dist Dx...absent

<u>Right Coronary Artery:</u>

  Prox RCA...70% discrete stenosis

  Mid RCA...is normal

  Dist RCA....50% tubular stenosis; distal to lesion, segment small

  R PDA....80% discrete stenosis

<u>Left Main Coronary Artery:</u>   Normal

<u>Left Anterior Descending:</u>

  Prox LAD.....50% diffuse disease

  Mid LAD...is normal

  Dist LAD...is normal

<u>Left Circumflex Artery:</u>

  Intermed...60% discrete stenosis; distal to lesion, segment small

<u>Assessment of Bypassability</u> of vessels with lesions 50%

  (based on the angiographic size and morphology of the distal vessel)

      RCA ....bypassability uncertain

      LAD............is bypassable

      Intermed..bypassability uncertain

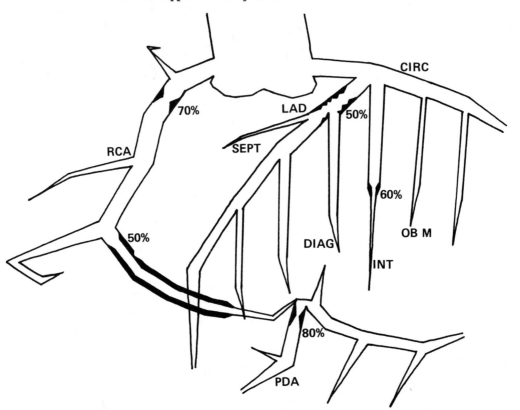

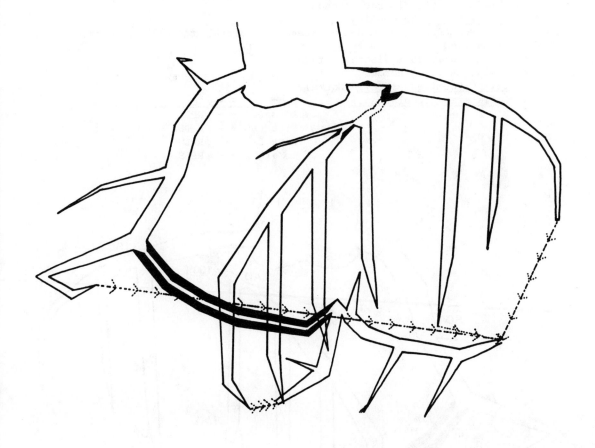

QUIZ #4. CORONARY ARTERIOGRAPHY

<u>Anatomy of native coronary arteries:</u>

  Dominance: Right

  LAD branches: Diag 1....large   Diag 2....large   Diag 3....large
                   Dist LAD..large

  Cx branches: Intermed..absent
                  ObMarg 1..large   ObMarg 2...small
                  Dist Cx...small

<u>Right Coronary Artery:</u>

  Dist RCA...90% tubular stenosis

<u>Left Main Coronary Artery:</u>

  LMCA.....50% discrete stenosis

<u>Left Anterior Descending</u>

  Prox LAD...100% discrete stenosis; distal to lesion, segment poorly
visualized

  Mid LAD ....90% discrete stenosis

  Dist LAD...is normal

<u>Left Circumflex Artery:</u> Normal

<u>Collateral Circulation:</u>

From -- -- --	To
Ac Marg ---	RPLS
Dist LAD ---	R PDA
Dist Cx ---	RPLS
ObMarg 1 ---	RPLS

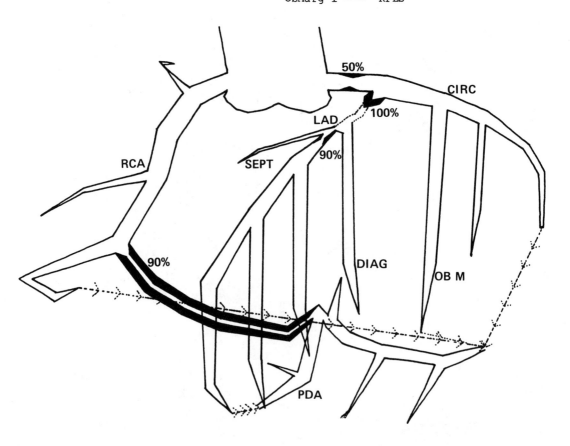

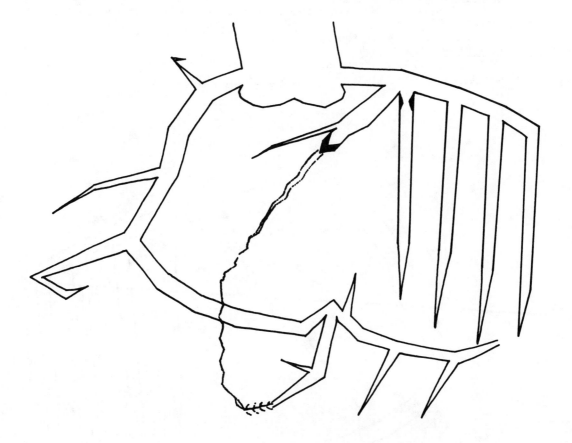

QUIZ #5. CORONARY ARTERIOGRAPHY

<u>Anatomy of native coronary arteries:</u>
Dominance: Right
LAD branches:
                Dist LAD..large
Cx branches: Intermed..large
                ObMarg 1..large   ObMarg 2 large   ObMarg 3 large
                Dist Cx...absent
<u>Right Coronary Artery:</u> Normal
<u>Left Main Coronary Artery:</u> Normal
<u>Left Anterior Descending:</u>
  Mid LAD..100% discrete stenosis; distal to lesion, segment poorly visualized
  Dist LAD is poorly visualized
<u>Left Circumflex Artery:</u>
  Intermed...70% discrete stenosis
<u>Collateral Circulation:</u>   <u>From -- -- -- To</u>
                      R PDA   ---   Dist LAD

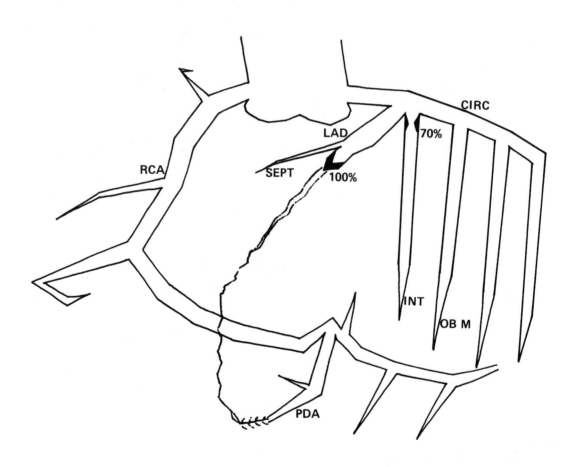

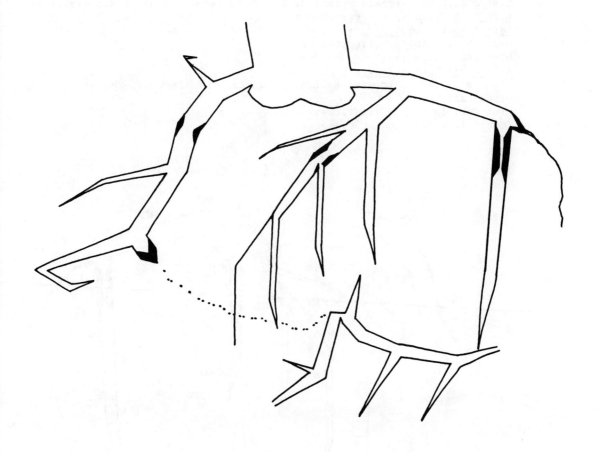

QUIZ #6.   CORONARY ARTERIOGRAPHY

Anatomy of native coronary arteries:

Dominance: Right

LAD branches: Diag 1....medium....   Diag 2....small   Diag 3....small
                Dist LAD..small

Cx branches: Intermed..absent
                ObMarg 1..large
                Dist Cx...small

Right Coronary Artery:

Prox RCA...50% discrete stenosis

Mid RCA...is normal

Dist RCA..100% discrete stenosis; distal to lesion, segment not visualized

Left Main Coronary Artery: Normal

Left Anterior Descending:

Mid LAD .....50% tubular stenosis

Dist LAD.....is small

Left Circumflex Artery:

Mid Cx...100% discrete stenosis; distal to lesion, segment poorly
visualized

Dist Cx...is poorly visualized

ObMarg 1....85% tubular stenosis

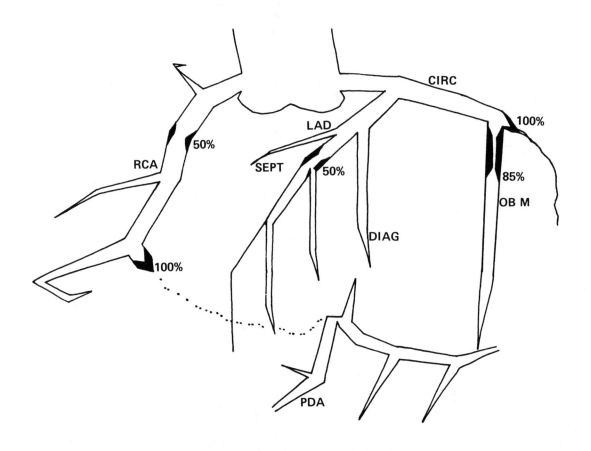

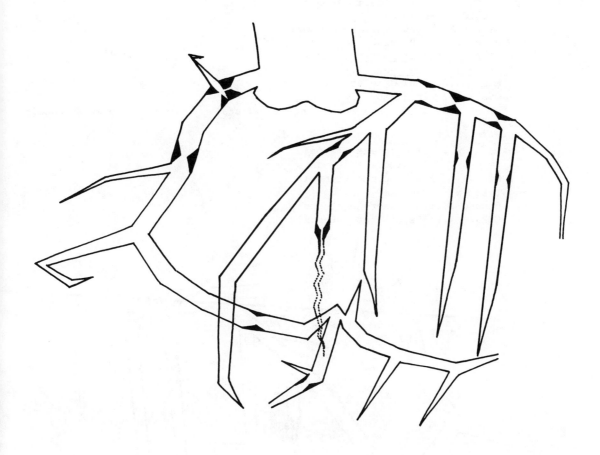

QUIZ #7.   CORONARY ARTERIOGRAPHY

<u>Anatomy of native coronary arteries:</u>

  Dominance: Right

  LAD branches: Diag 1....large   Diag 2....large

                Dist LAD..large

  Cx branches: Intermed..absent

                ObMarg 1..large   ObMarg 2..large

                Dist Cx....small

<u>Right Coronary Artery:</u>

  Prox RCA...90% discrete stenosis

             80% discrete stenosis

  Mid RCA...is normal

  Dist RCA ...50% discrete stenosis

  R PDA.......50% discrete stenosis

<u>Left Main Coronary Artery:</u> Normal

<u>Left Anterior Descending:</u>

  Mid LAD.....50% discrete stenosis

  Dist LAD...is normal

  Diag 2.....95% discrete stenosis; distal to lesion, segment poorly visualized

<u>Left Circumflex Artery:</u>

  Prox Cx...30% discrete stenosis

           95% discrete stenosis

  Mid Cx   95% discrete stenosis

  Dist Cx   is normal

  ObMarg 2...30% discrete stenosis

  ObMarg 1...30% discrete stenosis

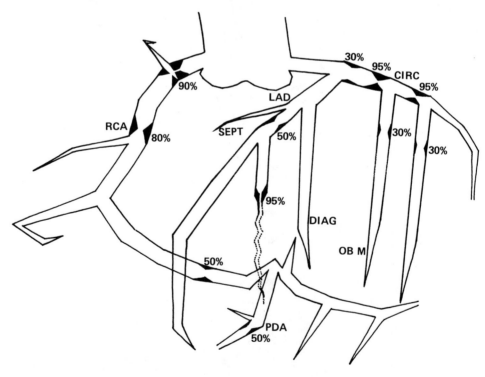

INDEX

Page numbers in italics indicate illustrations; page numbers followed by a t indicate tables.

Tachycardias, superventricular, 89
Thrombosis, *56, 78,* 83, *86, 98, 100*
   peripheral arterial, 85*t,* 87–88
Thrombus. *See* Thrombosis
Transluminal angioplasty, 96, *97*
Tricuspid valve, 4
T waves, *77, 79*

Valium (Diazepam), used to reduce anxiety, 83, 84
Valve competency, 62
Valves, cardiac
   aortic, 4, 18, 58, *60, 61,* 62
   calcification of, 58
   mitral, 4, 58, *59, 61,* 62
   motion of, 58, *59, 60*

pulmonary, 4
tricuspid, 4
Valve surgery, 18, 19*t*
Vasovagal reaction, 85*t,* 89
   symptoms of, 89
   treatment of, 89
Vena cava
   inferior, 2, *3*
   superior, 2, *3*
Ventricle
   left (*see* Left ventricle)
   right, 2, *3,* 4
Ventricular dysfunction, 85*t,* 88, 90
Ventricular fibrillation, 88
Ventriculography, 4, 51–62
   arrhythmias during, 78

catheters used in, 76, 78
extrasystoles during, 78
injection speed for, 78
injection volume for, 78
as prognostic tool, 4, 51
Vessel overlap, in angiograms, 16, 26, 34, 38
Vessel spasm, 82, 84, 86
Vieussens ring, 48

Wall motion, of left ventricle, 53, 54–55
   paradoxical, 55
Wall thickness, of left ventricle, 58
Wexler graft catheters, *70, 71, 76*